WITHOUT
MORAL
LIMITS

UPDATED EDITION

WITHOUT
MORAL
LIMITS

WOMEN, REPRODUCTION, AND MEDICAL TECHNOLOGY

DEBRA EVANS

CROSSWAY BOOKS • WHEATON, ILLINOIS
A DIVISION OF GOOD NEWS PUBLISHERS

Cover design: Liita Forsyth

Cover photo: The Stock Market

First printing of revised edition 2000

Printed in the United States of America

Library of Congress Cataloging-in-Publication Data
Evans, Debra.
    Without moral limits : women, reproduction, and medical technology / Debra Evans.—Rev. ed.
      p.   cm.
    Includes bibliographical references and index.
    ISBN 1-58134-201-2
    1. Human reproductive technology—Moral and ethical aspects. I. Title.
RG133.5.E89   2000
176—dc21   00-010334
                                            CIP

15	14	13	12	11	10	09	08	07	06	05	04	03	02	01	00
15	14	13	12	11	10	9	8	7	6	5	4	3	2	1	

For my daughters and granddaughters,
Joanna White and Katherine Evans,
Abigail and Makenzie White

The endless cycle of idea and action,

Endless invention, endless experiment,

Brings knowledge of motion, but not of stillness;

Knowledge of speech, but not of silence;

Knowledge of words, and ignorance of the Word.

All our knowledge brings us nearer to our ignorance,

All our knowledge brings us nearer to death,

But nearness to death no nearer to God.

Where is the Life we have lost in living?

Where is the wisdom we have lost in knowledge?

Where is the knowledge we have lost in information?

The cycles of Heaven in twenty centuries

Bring us farther from God and nearer to the Dust.

—T. S. ELIOT, FROM *THE ROCK, CHORUS I*

CONTENTS

PREFACE

Strangely enough, the incident that sparked the desire to write this book was an appointment I had at a dental college—an odd place to start a research project on reproductive medicine, I must admit. As a volunteer in the University of Nebraska-Lincoln Dental School's board exams, I hadn't realized that in exchange for receiving a free gold filling I would end up spending two full days as a senior student's model mouth.

Needless to say, when a break arrived for lunch that first morning, I had little desire to head for the cafeteria, so I visited the campus library next door instead. While searching through rows of bookshelves in the human development stacks, I noticed a book curiously titled *Marriage and Family in the Year 2020*. One of the editors, Lester Kirkendall, was a name I had become familiar with while teaching sex education at the university. (Kirkendall had been a cofounder of the Sex Information and Education Council of the United States, or SIECUS, the group responsible for introducing situation ethics and values clarification into sex education programs around the nation.) *Interesting*, I can remember thinking. *I wonder where Kirkendall hopes our culture will be when this generation's grandchildren reach adulthood.*

I checked the book out and immediately retreated to the lobby of the college to wait until the dental boards resumed. The contributors to the book, I discovered, had written their essays as if they were professors already living in the next century, reminiscing about how the American family had moved beyond a traditional belief system to a more "fully human" philosophy of life. Looking up Kirkendall's piece, "The Transition from Sex to Sexuality and Intimacy," I found these introductory statements:

> Explaining to persons living today, in 2020, how sensuality and intimacy were regarded in earlier centuries presents problems. To begin with, the language used in the past two centuries to describe these qualities has changed. Over time, various words and phrases have become obsolete, forgotten, abandoned; new

ones have taken their place. So we must begin our discussion by examining these language changes.

Even as recently as a century ago, the primary, and also the only morally acceptable use of the sensual organs, then known as the genitals, was to produce offspring. . . . Since children came as a result of joining the female/male sensual organs, these were referred to as the "reproductive organs." But as children became economically less profitable and the reproductive emphasis diminished, penile-vaginal coupling was used less and less for procreation, and the term "reproductive organs" was almost completely dropped. It was then that the term "sex organs" came into being. But that term is now seldom heard. About the only time "sex" is used is when someone inquires as to the gender of a newly-lifed, or newly-delivered child (formerly said to be "newborn"), but for most of us even that information has relatively little significance. Female and male have become so similar in their life patterns that no one cares much about sex membership in the old-fashioned sense. . . . We are all human beings first, female or male later.[1]

Then Kirkendall cites a note of warning (promise?) from someone whose name immediately recalls the not-so-distant sixties— Marshall McLuhan. A piece he had cowritten with George Leonard, predictably titled *The Future of Sex,* had appeared in *Look* magazine nearly twenty years prior to my date with the dentist:

Sex as we think of it may soon be dead. Sexual concepts, ideals, and practices already are being altered almost beyond recognition. . . . What it will mean to be a boy or a girl, man or woman, husband or wife, male or female, may come as one of the great surprises the future holds for us.[2]

Eliminating the biological differences through muting, altering, or obliterating the unique reproductive functions of men and women will mean the betrayal of marriage and the family—not their future, I thought. What is happening to women? What will happen to tomorrow's children? Where will we be once we finally get to where today's attitudes are taking us?

Glancing up at the clock, I noticed I had twenty minutes left before resuming my day-long adventure in dentistry. I read through Kirkendall's list of the seven social trends he predicts will change the face of sexuality:

- increased control over reproductive processes
- increasing acceptance of sensuality and intimacy
- harmonizing intimacy with other life experiences
- acceptance of equalitarian ways of attaining gender identity
- a shift in behavior models
- a rounded life
- emphasis on rationality in decision-making

He then describes the cultural abandonment of all historic sexual taboos. Incest, the need for privacy, sanctions against public self-stimulation, and rules against sexual interaction between people of widely differing ages, he explains, have all been dropped. Sex education has been replaced with "sensual intimacy education." All of this is presented as desirable, normal, wanted. (By whom?) I could not help wondering what such a society would be like, knowing what our current level of reproductive confusion has already unleashed upon us.

In his discussion of "The Process-Oriented Versus the Act-Oriented Value System," Kirkendall concludes:

> The integration of sensuality and intimacy into the whole of life has moved us toward different moral/value concepts. A century ago the above heading would have been "*The Existing Moral Code.*" People were praised or condemned by their compliance with a rigid and limiting code of prescribed acts. At that time, the code centered heavily on sensual/intimacy activities. The intent was to ban any relating which might lead to pregnancy, to sexually transmitted diseases, or result in pleasure. This essentially barred any personal, private, or group sensual activity, except for a physical connection (i.e. intercourse) in which the possibility of procreation was fully accepted. Anything else was a perversion. But as the rigid code relaxed, new concepts evolved. At the same time vocabulary was altered: perversions became abnormalities, abnormalities

became deviancies, deviancies became variations, variations became options, options became preferences, preferences became choices, and choices became life-enhancing experiences. With these developments came diversity and a growing concern with values geared toward building caring and responsible relationships.[3]

In one paragraph Dr. Kirkendall dismisses centuries of cross-cultural wisdom as an "existing moral code!" Why is he so eager to sacrifice the sanctity of marriage to a me-centered morality that has inflicted intense pain and suffering upon so many lives? What human toll does chastity reap in comparison to widespread sexual addiction?

With this, my lunch break ended. I spent the afternoon under the influence of Novocain, tilted back beneath the softly filtered beams of an examining light, reflecting upon what the term "sexual revolution" actually means. I began thinking in larger terms about how some current assumptions regarding lovemaking, procreation, and assisted reproductive technologies can diminish women's God-designed dignity.

Later I read more of Kirkendall's book. I learned about the mechanization of reproduction, artificial wombs, and the cryopreservation of human embryos, of the "final liberation" of women from their "biological destiny" and its complementary effect upon men. I often wept at the vision that emerged before me, not wanting to believe my eyes, and eventually I gathered over 6,000 pages of documentation to substantiate my concerns.

Concentrating on key journal articles written by physicians and scientists, I present to you evidence that this revolution was successfully manipulated and exploited by medicine during the twentieth century, leading to unregulated human experimentation and rapid proliferation of assisted reproductive technologies (ARTs) in industrialized Western nations. A new ethic now pervades what were formerly known as the healing arts. It is already affecting all of our lives.

INTRODUCTION

In the Metropolitan Museum of Art hangs a little-known Renaissance painting that is easy to miss unless you are specifically looking for it. Rarely pondered for its theme or composition, the subtly shaded canvas must vie for attention with dozens of world-famous pieces. Still, this unusual portrait makes a powerful statement. Time has not changed the beauty of the woman represented here, nor has it diminished the value of her message. She seems to be waiting to teach those willing to stop and look.

Clothed in a long, loosely gathered rose-toned dress, a beige shawl softly draped around her auburn hair and shoulders, she appears almost casual; she is elegant, relaxed, and open with her body. No harsh edges obscure the smooth contours of her features. Kindness glimmers in the radiance of her smile.

But something more is going on in this picture. Next to the woman's heart reclines a naked toddler, calmly sucking at her breast, while another infant peacefully dozes in her lap. A third child at her right shoulder has captured his mother's attention. Their eyes meet as she seems to reassure him that he will be next to nurse. Her steady presence and ease of posture impart a transcendent dignity to the scene. The painting is titled *Charity*.

Charity? Surrounded by the needs of several infants, prepared to nurse two in rapid succession, this gentle matron affronts our modern notions of sexuality and procreative freedom. If such a picture were painted of this woman today, people would be offended. Critics would no doubt denounce the preposterous presentation of three nursing toddlers. Since breasts are no longer viewed as an integral symbol of comfort and compassion, it would be challenging to understand this woman in less than overtly sexual terms.

The meaning of women's breasts has been fundamentally altered since the 1930s in the Western industrialized nations, their reproductive role having been almost entirely exchanged for the erotic as a cultural symbol. Consequently, "boobs" are featured in advertisements for everything from deodorants to diet soda, but not in portraits of nursing babies. Visitors from third-world countries remark about the recreational fixation our country has with this part of the anatomy, perplexed at why so much national attention is geared toward certain sets and sizes of attractively displayed mammary glands.

Considering how quickly this aspect of women has been sexualized and subsequently exploited—all in the space of just one generation, in no small part due to the widespread use of bottled infant formula—it is not unreasonable to wonder what effects new reproductive technologies and changing attitudes about human sexuality will have upon other expressions of women's procreative experiences in successive generations.

In the same way that bottle-feeding made breastfeeding biologically optional, widespread cultural acceptance of contraception, abortion, sterilization, and other counter-reproductive technologies have rendered the womb optional as well. Unless a woman chooses to be pregnant, it is now the norm to view fertility itself as merely a peripheral aspect of female sexuality, an accessory feature to be turned on and off at will, an ofttimes irritating component of gender identity. In other words, procreation is no longer considered a key biological/emotional/social/spiritual component of a married woman's creative existence.

After the popularization of oral contraceptives in the 1960s, it took less than twenty years for sterility to become more acceptable than fertility, a vacant womb more valued than a pregnant one. "The 1960s brought sex without procreation; the 1980s brought procreation without sex," explains attorney Lori Andrews, an ARTs legal expert.[1] Our social consciousness has moved closer to the reproductive reality of Aldous Huxley's *Brave New World* than we might like to think.

Not all women, however, accept these cultural and technological changes as a step forward for humanity. I, for one, am grieved that the "blessings of the breast and womb"[2] —nursing and childbearing—are no longer regarded as cultural symbols of love and strength and generosity. I am grieved that a mother nursing her young children has become an antiquated metaphor for charity and compassion, that flowing breast milk is commonly regarded as an embarrassment rather than a gift.

I am grieved that our society has become increasingly captivated by sexual exploitation and pornography while growing hostile toward women's normal and natural reproductive design. I am grieved that hundreds of thousands of women will lose their fertility this year, victims of a worldwide epidemic of sexually transmitted infections such as chlamydia, gonorrhea, and HPV (human papilloma virus). I am especially grieved that some of these women will also lose their lives.

It is tragic that more than one in every five babies in the United States is born by cesarean section, delivered by surgeons through incisions in their mother's abdomens instead of being actively birthed by the women themselves, with at least half of these operations deemed unnecessary by various public health experts. I am grieved when women feel that their best choice is to open their wombs to physicians' cannulas and curettes rather than to the life-giving act of birth. And I am grieved at the transfer of lovemaking and conception to the medical clinic and the research laboratory where a woman's body becomes an apparatus and her eggs subject to search and seizure.

The question that keeps haunting me is this: If the biological integrity of woman continues to be invaded, altered, and separated from her soul, what will happen to the children? When the appointed guardians of new life are removed, civilization can become coolly efficient and calculated toward its weakest citizens. When family bonds fracture, social programs attempt to replace family nurture and traditional wisdom; substitutes and surrogates are hired to fulfill maternal responsibilities. The betrayal of woman results in commercialization of the natural processes that create and maintain the basic bonds of life.

Children are not commodities to be bought and sold—they are God's precious gifts, to be accepted, protected, and cared for without discrimination on the basis of sex, size, DNA code, or developmental condition.

We are in danger of becoming a culture that neglects this fundamental human truth if we no longer collectively value the uniqueness of man and woman or the life created between them. We sometimes think we can buy/design/produce/acquire anything for the right price—including children. As a culture, we have not reached consensus on ethical issues surrounding conception and the prenatal period. Consequently, techniques that manipulate women's wombs, eggs, and offspring flourish. The development and proliferation of ARTs—too often based on a thirst for profit and the opportunity for research, discovery, and the pioneering of even better techniques, as later chapters will show—is taking place at breakneck speed without moral limits.

Birth, death, and even conception itself are increasingly relegated to the dominion of medical science, thus placing our faith, as Eliot noted, "farther from God and nearer to the Dust." The chemical, surgical, and cultural alteration of human sexuality and procreation is symbolic of this process—advance warning of what may come.

It is as if someone had repeatedly stolen into the art museum and vandalized the painting of the charitable, compassionate figure, one step at a time, erasing first her breasts, severing her vital connection to the children. The texture of the woman's skin subtly changes. A variety of interesting objects appear in the background and then move to a position of prominence in the portrait. Infants begin to disappear from the surface of the canvas, eventually leaving only a solitary figure.

With a few more strokes of the brush, the transformation is complete: A new image has appeared, wholly representative of sexual autonomy, reproductive choice, and personal freedom. The openhearted embodiment of charity has vanished. Without breasts or womb, a woman from the late twentieth century gazes with longing into the distance.

Chapter One

Lab-Oriented Conceptions and *Mis*-conceptions: The Early History of Egg Harvesting and Embryo Experimentation

The term "reproductive revolution" is not mere hyperbole. . . . Like Caesar crossing the Rubicon, there is no turning back from the technical control that we now have over human reproduction. The decision to have or not have children is, at some important level, no longer a matter of God and nature, but has been made subject to human will and technical expertise. It has become a matter of choice whether persons reproduce now or later, whether they overcome infertility, whether their children have certain genetic characteristics, or whether they use their reproductive capacity to produce tissue for transplant or embryos and fetuses for research.[1]

—JOHN A. ROBERTSON, *CHILDREN OF CHOICE*

These are not perverted men in white coats doing nasty experiments on human beings, but reasonable scientists carrying out perfectly justifiable research.[2]

—*NATURE*

The idea of man's accelerating control over his own reproductive capacities has come of age.[3]

—ROBERT T. FRANCOEUR, *UTOPIAN MOTHERHOOD*

In the earliest weeks of prenatal development, each tiny female embryo contains stem cells that later organize into two small clumps of tissue high in the fetal abdomen near the kidneys. At the time of birth a complete supply of about half a million immature eggs will have formed in these twin almond-shaped clusters. When the girl reaches puberty, all but approximately 10,000 ova will have degenerated. When she reaches fifty, most will have disappeared.

Over a span of about thirty-five years, from menarche until menopause, only 400 to 500 eggs are stimulated by hormones to develop within a woman's ovaries.

During the preovulatory phase of the menstrual cycle, fifteen to twenty ova are brought to the brink of ripening. In most cases, only a single egg bursts forth each month from its fluid-filled sac lying within one of the ovaries. A mature egg, once released from this ripened follicle, is actually quite fragile, requiring continual nourishment and protection as it enters the fallopian tube and begins its long journey toward the womb. This nurture is provided by a billowy, heaped-up mass of "nurse cells," called cumulus cells, that escape from the follicle along with the egg. After leaving the ovary, an ovum is receptive to fertilization for only twelve to twenty-four hours.

As it passes into the pelvic cavity, the liberated egg is then literally picked up by the fringed fimbria ("fingers") at the entrance of the fallopian tube. Here the egg is greeted by thousands of continuously beating hairlike filaments called cilia, which create a constant current toward the womb. The egg is thus propelled forward and cleansed of its cumulus cells; rhythmic muscular contractions within the oviduct's wall contribute to the one-way path the ovum is compelled to travel as well.

Until recently it was only here, in the distant portion of an oviduct, that the fate of a minuscule egg could be decided. Deep within the warmth of a woman's fallopian tube, sheltered protectively under layers of skin and fat and muscle, the ovum undergoing fertilization merges with a single sperm, one of several million released during an episode of lovemaking. The transmission of life from one generation to another had never happened in any other way. A woman's body held all the wonders and mysteries of her child's conception.

In the history of science, the twentieth century will be remembered for many things, but among the most significant, the disconnection of life's beginnings from the mysterious intimacy of sexual love will be ranked right along with the Manhattan Project, mass-produced antibiotics, and the discovery of DNA.

Two Historic Hunts for Human Eggs

The transfer of conception from the center of human sexuality to the control of third-party producers is built upon a forty-year legacy of clandestine egg hunts and extralegal embryo experimentation. By the time the first "test-tube baby" was born by cesarean section in 1978, hundreds of eggs had already been surgically removed from women's ovaries and reproductive tracts, inseminated in petri dishes, and examined with exacting detail under microscopes. Without this fundamental research, the generation of human life in the laboratory would never have been possible.

Of all the scientific searches for human ova conducted to date, two stand out—the fifteen-year egg hunt performed by obstetrician-gynecologists John Rock and Arthur Hertig in the United States and the studies of geneticist Robert Edwards and obstetrician-gynecologist (ob/gyn) Patrick Steptoe in England. Many more experiments using human ova have been (and are still being) conducted,[4] but only these four research pioneers were bold enough to publish detailed personal accounts of their work.[5]

Before 1938, the year the Rock-Hertig project began, very little was known about the intricate mechanisms involved in sexual reproduction. It was not until 1827 that the existence of a human egg was discovered. Another sixteen years went by before it was clearly demonstrated that a sperm actually enters an ovum during conception. Only in 1875 was it shown that fertilization takes place when the nucleus of the sperm joins with that of the ovum. The two sex hormones produced by the ovaries, estrogen and progesterone, were not discovered until 1929 and 1934. It was at this point in history that Dr. Rock and Dr. Hertig entered the race to discover additional secrets about early human development.

The site of the team's exploration of fertility and embryology was the privately endowed Free Hospital for Women in Brookline, Massachusetts, an affiliate of Harvard Medical School. Founded in

1875, the hospital admitted only poor women. The patients could not be charged for their medical care, nor were the physicians who worked there paid a fee. Charitable contributions covered all the costs of the elective gynecological surgery performed at the Free Hospital. The medical services were offered in quiet, elegant surroundings in a French-style estate house located in a beautiful riverside glen on four acres of land outside Boston. The "Free" was quite large and well-equipped for that era, with fifty in-patient beds, three operating rooms, modern X-ray equipment, fully equipped laboratories, and the first intensive-care recovery room in the country.

In exchange for their professional services, the Free Hospital for Women offered almost absolute research freedom to the physicians and medical students who worked there. John Rock's biographer explains the situation this way:

> During Rock's scientifically bountiful years there, the Free became something of a private research preserve for its princi-pal staffers, a cultured as well as competent clique of men also well versed in Harvard academic politics and content to remain aloof on their own protected turf. While medical insiders knew more or less what was going on in the research programs at the Free, the general public knew little of it.[6]

What exactly did some of the Free's little-known research entail? The harvesting of some 1,000 eggs from the dissected wombs, tubes, and ovaries of hundreds of hysterectomized patients. The artificial insemination of ova extracted from these organs with the sperm of medical students without the consent of the eggs' "donors." And strategically timed surgery scheduled to coincide with prospective patients' love lives and ovulatory cycles for the purpose of obtaining fresh, fertilized ova.

During this project nearly three dozen human beings in their earliest stages of life, found in women's tubes and uteri that had been removed by Dr. Rock, were painstakingly prepared and mounted for framing by Dr. Hertig and his dedicated coterie of lab-oratory technicians.

Conceptuses, Abortuses, or Human Waste?

The ethical implications of this research—lack of informed consent from participants, the performance of early abortions, human experimentation, and the exploitation of impoverished women—were dismissed by the two obstetrician-gynecologists. They worked for the good of science. "Induced abortions were illegal in Massachusetts, and the Free Hospital for Women was not running an abortion clinic," Hertig points out. "However, we and others were vitally interested in early human development."[7]

Potential ovum donors, most of whom were Catholics, had to meet very specific criteria in order to be considered for admission to the program. In addition to their need to have a hysterectomy, they were required to be "married and living with their husbands, intelligent, and to have demonstrated prior fertility by delivering at least three full-term pregnancies, and they had to be willing to record menstrual cycles and coitus without contraception."[8] This information was carefully recorded from postcards mailed to Dr. Rock's assistant, Miriam Menkin, in order to determine the scheduling of each operation.

The Pill, John Rock and the Church comments on the attitudes of the physicians toward their work:

> It unquestionably was a delicate ethical maneuver. Both Rock and Hertig thought about the ethical implications long and hard. Eventually, for both, it came down to "a necessary scientific endeavor using material that would have gone to waste but would not have been put to the use for which the Lord intended it." Neither Rock nor Hertig considered the conceptuses they hoped to find to be abortuses. At the few days to two or so weeks of development of the fertilized eggs, Hertig and Rock considered them undifferentiated bits of protoplasm, tiny gelatinous packets of human protein, destined to end up, undetected, in a surgical waste bin. . . .
>
> But the question hangs in the air. Couldn't the women have been instructed to refrain from marital intercourse and thereby eliminate any possibility of pregnancy at the time of surgery? Hertig vehemently maintained that they were not instructed *to* have intercourse, or *not* to, but only to record it if they did.[9]

Clearly, by their own admission the doctors were looking for "conceptuses"—conceived human beings undergoing their initial phases of embryonic development. "We were not doing abortions," Hertig insists, "but we hoped we would find [a fertilized] ovum."[10] By walking the fine line made possible by a lack of reliable means to detect pregnancy in its earliest stages, this approach was morally defensible in the minds of these physicians.

But what about the mothers of the "conceptuses"? Since the pregnancies were never "confirmed" and none of the women had missed a period, Hertig stresses, "There was no way in God's world at that time of knowing whether they were pregnant or not. There were literally no tests."[11] Apparently, according to his way of thinking, what the women didn't know certainly wouldn't hurt them, and it would help the cause of science, not to mention the team of Rock and Hertig, a great deal.

Another question that remains is, how much of the surgery performed on these women was unnecessary? An article appearing in the *Journal of the American Medical Association* in 1952 reported the removal of 704 normal ovaries from 546 patients in the Los Angeles area.[12] "Our patients' faith and trust will be justified so long as we are professionally and intellectually honest with them and ourselves," wrote Dr. James C. Doyle.[13] Yet he admitted that the "unwarranted sacrifice of normal ovaries" was "not at all unusual" as demonstrated by the statistics he had carefully collected.[14] The report is especially significant because it is from exactly the same period of time that the hunt for human ova at the Free Hospital for Women was being conducted.

In 1948 John Rock and Arthur Hertig were presented the coveted American Gynecological Society Award for their groundbreaking work. At the award banquet the dynamic duo was affectionately dubbed "the ham and the egg."[15]

A Morula Named Dominic

Rock and Hertig's active search for women's unborn offspring during the first two weeks of prenatal life lasted from 1938 until 1953.

During this time Dr. Hertig managed to take thirty-four early embryos from Dr. Rock's unknowingly pregnant patients.

Inspecting the "specimens," as Hertig refers to the extracted organs, was accomplished by examining ovaries, flushing fallopian tubes, cutting over 200 wombs in half and carefully incising the uterine tissue while it was immersed at room temperature under a specially prepared fluid. "By tubal washing and this uterine technique," claims Hertig, "we obtained all the significant preimplanting stages of human development."[16]

Following this procedure, Dr. Hertig would then look over the uterus twice, both before and after applying a special fixative called Bouin's fluid to clarify the womb's surface. By this method Hertig was able to find embryos up to seventeen days of age nesting in the womb's lining. "Surprisingly, all the normal conceptuses were found implanted on the posterior wall of the uterus, whereas all those considered abnormal were located on the anterior wall," Dr. Hertig dryly reports in the *American Journal of Obstetrics and Gynecology*.[17]

Hertig recounts a favorite story from his work in an article he wrote:

> The following anecdote illustrates the interest in the project on the part of my house staff, the clinical house staff, and the visiting staff and faculty. During the 1946 World Series between the Boston Red Sox and the St. Louis Cardinals, in the eighth inning, Dominic DiMaggio (Red Sox centerfielder) hit a double that tied the game and the series. Of course, we (the Red Sox) went on to lose the series (and game) when Enos Slaughter stole home on his single, owing to Johnny Pesky's moment of indecision in throwing to home plate. Of importance to this tale is the fact that I found, at the moment of Dominic's double, an unimplanted nine-cell ovum that proved, like the series, to be a pathological one! As was the custom in those days, when early human ova (i.e., embryos) were rarely found, illustrated, and published, the finder's name was affixed to the specimen he or she discovered. Thus, this pathological nine-cell morula-ovum was appropriately named "Dominic." I found it the minute he hit his famous double against the left field wall of Fenway Park.[18]

The christened embryo was preserved for posterity and eventually placed on public display as Plate #47 in the Carnegie human embryology collection in Baltimore.

"I have been told by experts in in vitro fertilization that this series of naturally occurring human ova laid the foundation for their pioneering work in solving developmental aspects of human infertility," Dr. Hertig explains.[19]

It is from this small beginning that the new medicine of laboratory-oriented conception was born.

Nearly 800 Human Follicular Eggs Have Been Isolated

Whereas Arthur Hertig has the distinction of being the first to find and photograph a series of early human embryos, his partner John Rock is better known for other outstanding accomplishments in medicine. A famous actor as a Harvard undergraduate, Rock eventually became one of the most colorful figures in the history of obstetrics and gynecology.

As a practicing member of the Catholic church, Dr. Rock was the only Catholic among fifteen eminent Boston physicians to sign a petition circulated by Margaret Sanger's Birth Control League to repeal Massachusetts' birth control law. In 1936, soon after the "Rhythm Method" was propounded, he became the first in the United States to open a clinic teaching women of his denomination how to determine their monthly fertile period for the purpose of both attempting and avoiding pregnancy.

Undeterred by the doctrines of his faith concerning human sexuality, Rock pursued his scientific interest in gynecology with brilliant dedication. Throughout his entire career he remained at the forefront of medical bioengineering and infertility research—designing the now widely used vacuum aspirator/curettes to collect hundreds of uterine tissue samples for biopsy studies; spending several years measuring the electrical potential of women's vaginas in attempts to determine the timing of ovulation; testing the first synthetic materials to be used as replacements for damaged fallopian tubes; performing the earliest experiments with fertility drugs and sex hormones; and pioneering techniques now used in artificial insemination—the collection, freezing, and storage of sperm.

Dr. Rock was also a renowned speaker and writer. Among his most memorable contributions was a landmark article on human ovulation for the prestigious *New England Journal of Medicine* in 1941. In 1949, in the same journal, another of his remarkable papers was published: "The Physiology of Human Conception." Rock's greatest achievement came just over a decade after this article was printed, on May 11, 1960. His work with biologist Gregory Pincus regarding the influence of sex hormones on women's fertility resulted in the federal government's final approval of the first oral contraceptive.

To this long list of obstetrical and gynecological "firsts," the man who would become known as "the father of the Pill" desired to establish himself as the first physician to accomplish the extraordinary feat of test-tube conception. In 1944, along with his assistant Miriam Menkin, he wrote:

> First stages of cleavage [cell division] of the fertilized human egg have, as far as we know, never been reported, and while *in vitro* fertilization of tubal eggs of the rabbit has been described, we have found no record of such experiments with higher mammals. . . . Utilizing surgical material [i.e., women's ovaries] available at the Free Hospital for Women, we have, during the past six years, made numerous attempts to achieve *in vitro* fertilization and cleavage of human eggs obtained from ovarian tissue just prior to the expected time of ovulation.[20]

The process worked this way: Rock and Menkin would prepare hysterectomy patients at the Free by counseling them on how to keep an accurate record of their menstrual cycles prior to hospital admission. By operating close to the time of ovulation, they were able to maintain a supply of nearly ripe eggs for their trials of test-tube conception.

Throughout the research, Miriam Menkin would stand outside the operating room every Tuesday, holding a jar of sterile solution as she waited to collect ovaries, oviducts, and wombs. After carrying the excised organs to a small laboratory, Menkin would then flush the ovaries with the solution and drain the contents of each organ into a dish. Any eggs that she found were gently washed several times, transferred to a glass flask, and placed in blood taken from the egg "donor" prior to surgery. The ova would then be incubated in the blood at body temperature for twenty-four hours. When ripe eggs became available, a man who was willing to sell sperm to the hospital would be notified that his semen was needed.

John Rock coordinated and oversaw the semen collection portion of the program. By compiling a list of young interns from Harvard Medical School, Dr. Rock put together a group of men particularly eager to fulfill his requests. In exchange for a small fee, they were asked to masturbate and ejaculate semen samples into sterile containers. A special nonclinical atmosphere was created expressly for this purpose—a private cubicle lined with large posters of seductively posed nude women that Dr. Rock had brought back from Sweden to help "inspire the young men to action."[21] The job was quite simple in comparison to the role the women played in the project.

Between 1938 and 1944, nearly 800 human follicular eggs were isolated from ovaries during the course of the Menkin-Rock investigation in this way.[22] Of these, 138 were painstakingly observed for signs of prenatal development after exposure to medical students' fresh spermatozoa. The research was made possible by a grant from the Carnegie Corporation of New York.[23]

Mouse, Sheep, Cow, Pig, Rhesus Monkey . . . and Human Ovarian Oocytes

Without question, no one has contributed more to today's practice of in vitro fertilization (IVF) than Robert G. Edwards, a British scientist with a doctorate in animal genetics. In spite of reports published by John Rock and Miriam Menkin claiming that they had accomplished human fertilization in a test tube in 1944, it was Edwards who was the first to definitively achieve external human fertilization twenty-five years later.[24]

Nine years of intense research using human ova preceded this historic event. Edwards's story reveals the irresistible power science holds over researchers, nudging them step by step along the path of discovery. "If it can be done, it must be done" was the principle that propelled Edwards's research inexorably forward; the ethical implications of his work were considered unimportant in comparison to the knowledge to be gained by producing human life for examination in the laboratory.

In *A Matter of Life,* a book Edwards wrote with gynecologist Patrick Steptoe, we hear the voice of a man who had spent his entire career working with lab animals describe his initial shock at the harsh realities involved in hunting down human ova:

> Dissecting mice and rats, that was one thing. This was utterly different. Here, in the operating theater, I felt myself to be exactly what I was—a novice. I stood at the back, wearing a mask, careful not to touch anything. I obeyed all instructions to the letter. "Come forward now," directed Molly, and I came forward clutching my glass sterile pot—the receptacle for the precious bit of superfluous ovarian tissue.
>
> Two or three times a month I would be summoned to Edgware General Hospital. I was always impressed by Molly Rose's surgery. And, as I waited for her to call me forward, as I glimpsed the naked skin of another human being being cut and human blood spurting, the clamps applied, I sometimes questioned my right to be there. "What am I doing?" I asked myself. "Do I really have a place in this theater?" There on the operating table was a woman who had been ill, whom Molly hoped to make well again. . . . And I? I was there merely for some spare eggs, for a piece of ovary that had to be removed anyway and which I would take back to my safe laboratory bench in Mill Hill. . . .
>
> Now that I had a small but regular supply of human ova from Edgware—and elsewhere, for I had persuaded other gynecologists to bequeath me ovarian tissue also—I could plan my work.[25]

Unfortunately, Edwards's initial encounter with feelings of awe and shame while invading the privacy of Dr. Rose's anesthetized patients quickly wore off. After just five years, he had tracked down enough eggs to accumulate the necessary data to publish the details of human egg development in laboratory apparatus.[26] In his article titled "Maturation *In Vitro* of Mouse, Sheep, Cow, Pig, Rhesus Monkey, and Human Ovarian Oocytes," he identifies the major stumbling block imposed upon his work:

> The investigation of early development in many mammalian species is restricted by the difficulty of obtaining sufficient numbers of oocytes [eggs] and embryos at particular stages of development. . . .
>
> Only small pieces of ovary from patients undergoing surgery for various disorders were available, and the number of oocytes from any one piece were seldom sufficient to provide samples for examination after different periods of time.[27]

Nevertheless, Edwards's single-minded pursuit of human eggs and in vitro fertilization continued. His hunt took him from the British National Institute for Medical Research to the renowned Johns Hopkins Hospital in Baltimore, to a small group of gynecologists in North Carolina, and finally to a permanent academic post in the physiology department at Cambridge University in England.

From Surgical Patients to Infertile Couples

Robert Edwards's breakthrough arrived upon meeting a British gynecologist named Patrick Steptoe. To overcome difficulties in obtaining fresh human ova at exactly the right moment of maturation, Edwards realized it was essential to work with a physician who could combine regimens of hormone treatments with a simpler means of egg retrieval. Steptoe offered both. In his work with a large volume of patients at a branch of the National Health Service, Patrick Steptoe was the first physician in Great Britain to perfect the clinical use of a technique called laparoscopy.

By inserting a special stainless steel scope with its own light source into a woman's pelvic cavity, he could access the reproductive organs without major surgery. Through an inch-long incision made near the navel, and by expanding the abdominal cavity with carbon dioxide gas, diagnostic examinations and delicate surgery could be accomplished at a minimum of risk to the patient. The rate of postoperative discomfort and infection with laparoscopy was significantly less than with laparotomy, which involves a much larger incision, more extensive surgical repair, and a longer hospital stay.

After reading an article written by Steptoe about the new procedure, Edwards phoned him and told the gynecologist about his hopes of achieving in vitro fertilization. Steptoe was very receptive to the idea, having worked with the dilemma of infertility for a number of years, and he agreed to lend his expertise to Edwards's project. It was in this manner that the focus of IVF shifted from ovariectomy as a human egg source to the infertile women who willingly gave up their ova in hopes of becoming pregnant through in vitro fertilization.

Child Breeding in the Laboratory

As an animal geneticist, Edwards was not only interested in IVF's application to human infertility. Even though he knew infertile couples might eventually benefit from IVF, he was equally interested in the eugenic (selective breeding) potential and population control issues associated with extracorporeal (occurring outside the body) conception.

Edwards clearly understood that fertilizing human eggs in a laboratory setting does much more than bypass a pair of blocked fallopian tubes. Examination of chromosomes at the earliest stages of prenatal development permits an IVF technician to view an embryo's basic genetic makeup shortly after conception. Robert Edwards recognized this from the onset of his research. Virtually everything he has written on the subject describes the direct interrelationship between IVF and genetic diagnosis. In addition, his studies were financed by the Ford Foundation, a major financial backer of world population and eugenics-related research. Thus, it is highly doubtful that Edwards's grant source was primarily interested in the application of his work to the problem of human infertility.

Four years before he succeeded in producing the world's first test-tube conception, Edwards remarked:

It had occurred to me that, once the problem of human *in vitro* fertilization was solved, the sex of the embryos could be identified at a very early stage by examination of their chromosomes, and that it would be possible therefore to choose whether the mother gave birth to a girl or a boy. At first, animal husbandry would benefit. Farm animals could be induced to superovulate, their fertilized eggs removed, examined to see what sex they were, and only the ova of one or the other sex replaced into the womb of the mother animal. In man, certain diseases could perhaps be reduced.[28]

Today superovulation is regularly practiced in women as well as in sheep, pigs, and cattle. It is the standard practice of IVF clinics all over the world to synthetically induce multiple ovulation in women via hormone injections and medications prior to oocyte removal. The chromosome analysis of IVF embryos, predicted by Edwards, is already being utilized.[29] It is now possible, in fact, to use highly specific DNA "probes" to determine the sex of an eight-cell embryo and diagnose a variety of genetic disorders before selective transfer to a woman's womb via preimplantation diagnosis.[30]

Shortly after Robert Edwards had obtained large numbers of human eggs through his collaboration with infertility specialists at Johns Hopkins University, he concluded an article for *Scientific American* with these words on child breeding:

> We intend to continue these experiments; the ability to observe cleaving eggs could be of great medical and scientific value. . . . oocytes and embryos showing anomalies [defects] could be eliminated in favor of those developing normally. This achievement might one day permit some choice to be made in the type of offspring born to particular parents.[31]

In the first paper to announce Edwards's success with IVF, he begins by hailing the embryo's usefulness to science rather than with the progeny's intrinsic value or desirability to his or her parents. The message here is very clear about the importance of IVF to reproductive research:

The technique of maturing human oocytes *in vitro* after their removal from follicles provides many eggs for studies on fertilization. Their fertilization *in vitro* would yield a supply of embryos for research or clinical use, but in previous attempts the incidence was too low to be useful.[32]

Furthermore, Edwards proposes several novel ideas on how human embryos might specifically be used for the purpose of tissue harvesting and organ farming:

> Will we be able to extract the stem cells of various organs from the embryo, the precious foundation cells of all the body's organs, and then use them therapeutically? Will it ever be possible to use these cells to correct deficiencies in other human beings—to replace one deficient tissue with another that functions normally? For instance, will we be able to use the blood-forming tissue of an embryo to re-colonize defective blood-forming tissue in an adult or child? And will these notions be met with pursed lips and frowning faces?
>
> Perhaps the whole concept will fall to the ground and be proved to be a mistaken one in medical treatment. I doubt it, so much is on our side—the very foundation cells have been and will be again seen in our cultures and we know they are capable of displaying the initial signs of tissue differentiation. These same embryonic cells may offer us one further therapeutic advantage. They may one day be used [by cloning an embryo from a host "parent"] without having to worry about graft rejection such as we all know is associated with kidney, heart, and liver transplantations.
>
> Perhaps this whole approach may seem heartless to those who feel the embryo is a human being. . . . To grow fetuses to later stages of growth when they take a recognizable human shape and then extract their organs would be an utterly repugnant concept; but to obtain cell colonies from minute embryos useful in medicine for the alleviation of certain human disorders—is that not a legitimate target to aim at? It is a target that may be reached, should be reached, if we can understand the priceless secrets of those embryonic cells growing in our cultures.[33]

Were these statements simply the far-out fantasies of a Cambridge genetics professor—or the accurate predictions of the twentieth century's foremost international expert on human ectogenesis?

What in fact did Robert Edwards do with the dozens of embryos he created in the lab before the first was transferred to a woman's womb?

Were women who gave their eggs to Edwards accurately informed of the experimentation their offspring were involved in?

Is similar research still going on today with spare embryos obtained from the artificial insemination of women's eggs?

This final story gives some of the answers to these questions.

Bob's and Barry's Babies: Success at Last

Unbeknownst to their mother, the first children to be conceived in vitro were fathered by Robert G. Edwards and his Cambridge associate Barry D. Bavister. In March 1968 Edwards was able to get one final batch of fresh ova from a patient operated on by Dr. Rose. "This was the last piece of ovarian tissue that I was to obtain from Edgware General hospital," recalls Edwards. "It yielded me twelve human eggs."[34]

After ripening the eggs for thirty-six hours in a culture concocted by Bavister, the two men ejaculated their semen into collection bottles, washed their sperm by spinning them in a centrifuge, and poured the fluid into the culture medium where the eggs waited. Ten hours later, this is what Edwards found as he peered at the culture through a high-powered microscope:

> I held my breath. A spermatozoon was just passing into the first egg. We examined and re-examined it and there was no doubt. Marvelous. An hour later, we looked at the second egg. Yes, there it was, the early stages of fertilization. A spermatozoon had entered the egg without any doubt—we had done it. "Yes," I said softly.[35]

We can be certain that the woman from whom these eggs were taken had absolutely no idea that her ovary would be carried from the operating room, inspected for oocytes by a researcher at Cambridge University, and inseminated with the sperm of scientists. Nor did she know that her twelve ova would make history as the first human beings to be generated in a laboratory. The embryos created without her permission were methodically analyzed and painstakingly photographed by Edwards and Bavister for international publication.[36]

How many other ova have been extracted for use in research laboratories? Or inseminated with the sperm of strangers? How many more embryos have been created without their mother's knowledge? Mounted and framed for museum collections? Photographed in phase-contrast for scientific journals?

Some hospitals bury women's ovaries.[37] Considering what can happen to reproductive tissue these days, that seems a reasonable way to dispose of a woman's eggs.

Chapter Two

Sex in a Dish? In Vitro Fertilization and Embryo Transfer

Destruction of the natural means destruction of life. Knowledge and the will to live fall into disorder and confusion and are directed toward the wrong objects. The unnatural is the enemy of life.[1]

DIETRICH BONHOEFFER, ETHICS

In recent years stories of test-tube babies have been popular news items. But few Americans remember the names of John and Doris Del Zio, the first couple to attempt in vitro fertilization in the United States—and make national headlines in the process. Reflecting on this years later, Mrs. Del Zio explains, "I didn't do it to be the first; I did it because I wanted desperately to have our baby."[2] As the following story shows, it is this very desperation that made Doris the perfect target for experimental infertility treatment. In her article she shares the reasons behind her intense desire for a child:

> I found it difficult to understand the wide interest in my case. Who cares about me? I'm a nobody from Plattsburgh, N. Y. My father worked in a paper mill; my mother was a saleslady in a jewelry store and I never went to college. I went to airline-stewardess school, married for the first time at eighteen, had a baby girl at nineteen and separated from my husband at twenty.
>
> After my divorce, I worked at two jobs: as a receptionist for a doctor in the daytime and as a clerk in a grocery store at night. It was hard, but my daughter, Tammy, and I made it on our own.
>
> Then I met my present husband, Dr. John Del Zio, a dentist. Twenty-five years older than I, he had been separated from his wife for nine years. His compassion was immediately evident and all enveloping. He invited me out and, although divorced

women are fair game, I didn't have to fight him off. I felt comfortable with him and two years later we were married.

We had discussed having a large family and, from the moment I said "I do" in 1968, I couldn't wait to have another baby.[3]

Unfortunately, Doris Del Zio suffered a ruptured ovarian cyst on her honeymoon, requiring immediate surgery. The Del Zios then spent a full year trying to conceive. When it was discovered she wasn't ovulating regularly, Doris's physician put her on Clomid, a fertility drug he told her would greatly increase the likelihood of multiple pregnancy. Instead of producing twins or triplets, the drug brought on nausea, weight gain, and more painful cysts on her ovaries.

In February 1970 a diagnostic test called a hysterosalpingogram turned up a more serious problem. Doris's fallopian tubes were blocked. Her physician referred her to an infertility specialist, Dr. William J. Sweeney III, a professor of obstetrics and gynecology at Cornell University-New York Hospital. Further tests confirmed the tubal diagnosis. A procedure could be performed that might open her oviducts, Dr. Sweeney said, even though he could not guarantee success. Doris consented to the operation.

Like many infertile women, Doris had complete confidence in medicine's ability to come up with a solution to her problem. "I am a very simple person," she confesses. "If a faucet were broken, I'd have it fixed. If my tubes were blocked, I'd have them opened. I knew it wasn't that easy, but because I'd conquered polio when I was a little girl, I have great faith in science and medicine."[4]

In 1970 Dr. Sweeney performed a laparoscopy. But because of a childhood appendix operation and earlier surgery to remove her ruptured ovarian cyst, excessive scar tissue had developed inside Doris's abdomen. This made the tubal repair impossible. If her tubes could be opened at all, Dr. Sweeney told his client that a much more extensive and painful operation would be necessary.

For Doris there was no doubt the surgery was needed. She describes herself as a "fighter" and didn't mind undergoing additional surgery in order to become pregnant. From previous operations, she knew she was allergic to painkillers, and yet she remained positive about the operation. The reason, she said, was because "when I have hope, I can stand pain."[5] At this point Doris had already made a substantial emotional and financial investment in her battle against infertility. She was not ready give up the struggle as long as she had another option.

False Hopes and Unethical Human Experimentation

The operation was performed, and Doris conceived several months later in the autumn of 1970. Tragically, the pregnancy she had longed for ended in heartbreak. The baby miscarried at Christmastime.

By the following spring, Doris had not become pregnant and was anxious to resume medical treatment. She and John decided to fly to New York from their new home in Fort Lauderdale, Florida, to meet again with Dr. Sweeney. When he could offer no other therapy than attempting a second tubal reconstruction, Doris insisted on trying it.

In spite of the additional surgery and ongoing infertility treatment, pregnancy continued to elude the Del Zios. They attempted artificial insemination, with no results. In the meantime, additional cysts and adhesions had formed on Doris's reproductive organs. The likelihood that she would ever be pregnant again diminished.

Then she developed gall bladder problems in the fall of 1971—yet another medical crisis. "I was utterly miserable," she remembers. "My abdomen now looked like a road map, and my insides were a mass of adhesions. Sometimes they were so painful that I just couldn't straighten up. John felt that I had gone through enough, mentally and physically. I knew that, financially, he'd been through enough too."[6]

As with so many infertile couples today, the Del Zios continued to seek their physician's help in spite of the toll infertility treatment was taking. Doris traveled to see Dr. Sweeney again in April 1972. This time, however, he finally told her that she would not be able to conceive another child.

After two and a half painful years, countless office visits and exams, dozens of diagnostic procedures, risky hormone therapy, a laparoscopy, two tubal surgeries, the removal of her gall bladder, and a miscarriage, Doris was almost willing to give up her quest for conception. Facing Dr. Sweeney across his desk, she clearly remembers her reaction to hearing she couldn't become pregnant and to the strange piece of news that followed:

> Although his office was full of patients, he took the time to show me stacks of charts of women who had problems similar to mine. I cried all over his office. I was angry at medicine and science in general. "If they can get a man on the moon, why can't they let me get pregnant by bypassing my dumb little fallopian tubes?" I asked.
>
> It was a long time ago but I can still see him sitting behind his desk, his white coat all starched, his telephone with its innumerable buttons silent. He must have told his secretary to hold his calls.
>
> After my outburst he asked, "Have you read any articles about *in vitro* fertilization?"
>
> I hadn't. It was the first time I had heard the expression.
>
> "It's a way of getting pregnant without using the fallopian tubes," he explained. "But it has only been done with animals."[7]

One can easily imagine how Dr. Sweeney's words must have sounded to a woman who had endured so much in hope of giving birth to another child. Across the Atlantic, Patrick Steptoe and Robert Edwards had already discovered that infertile women with damaged oviducts were ideal candidates for experiments with in vitro fertilization. Now Doris Del Zio was about to become the first American woman to test the procedure. By her own account, Doris apparently believed IVF might produce a viable embryo capable of implanting in her uterus. The technique, however, had not yet been thoroughly studied in animals.

In June 1972 Doris had her third—and last—surgery in an attempt to repair her fallopian tubes. During the operation, Dr. Sweeney removed some of Doris's eggs and sent them along with a sample of John's sperm for a trial run at in vitro fertilization.

The man pioneering the procedure was Dr. Landrum Shettles, a physician-researcher at New York City's Columbia-Presbyterian

Hospital. Like Robert Edwards, Shettles had been conducting research on IVF with women's eggs since the 1950s.[8] But there was a significant difference between the two technicians. Shettles's work on external fertilization in humans had never been fully accepted by the international scientific community. Claiming that he had achieved IVF as early as 1955, Shettles had failed to sufficiently document his purported success through detailed photographs and descriptions of his research, as Edwards had done.

Nevertheless, the Del Zios' trial of IVF apparently worked; Dr. Sweeney informed the Del Zios there had been a "take." He told them they could try external fertilization if Doris couldn't conceive in the months following her third tubal operation. By December 1972, she still wasn't pregnant. The Del Zios were ready to go ahead with IVF.

"John supported me, but I was the driving force," admits Doris. "It took a year of mental, physical, and financial planning. We would have begged, borrowed, and mortgaged everything for a June hospitalization."[9]

The Del Zios flew to New York City in September 1973. Doris was in the operating room for over ten hours while her eggs were harvested. When she awoke from her anesthetic in the recovery room, she saw Dr. Sweeney standing at her bedside.

"We did well. We got the eggs," Doris remembers him telling her. She also adds:

> I was in great pain, but he was giving me hope.
>
> When I came down to my room, John had told me that he had taken the eggs to Dr. Shettles and all was well.
>
> The next day, although I still had a tube in my nose and an IV in my arm, I was happy. We talked about names for the baby.
>
> Later that afternoon, a nurse came in and told John that there was a call for him at the nurses' station. When John came back, he acted sort of funny. He didn't look me in the eye when he said, "Dr. Shettles called Dr. Sweeney and told him that the eggs weren't fertilizing."
>
> But I *knew* that the eggs had fertilized; there was something inside me that was sure.[10]

Later that evening, Dr. Shettles phoned Doris, saying over and over again, "I'm so sorry. I'm so sorry." It was the first time she had spoken to him.

Alone in her room, she listened to Landrum Shettles explain what had happened to her ova. When Shettles's supervisor, Dr. Raymond Vande Wiele, found out what had taken place, he stopped the IVF procedure by destroying the sterility of the eggs. The Del Zios later sued Vande Wiele, the hospital, and Columbia University for $1.5 million.

Defense attorneys argued that the procedure was dangerous and experimental—a fair and accurate portrayal considering the evidence. After hearing Doris recount her tragic story, the jury decided in favor of the Del Zios and their ill-fated offspring, awarding them $50,000 for the destruction of their embryos. (In retrospect, the case seems especially important in light of the Supreme Court's *Roe v. Wade* decision earlier in 1973.) The case continued to influence public policy, putting a halt to all federal research grants for the study of human in vitro fertilization in 1975, a moratorium that was not lifted until soon after President Clinton's 1992 inauguration.

Was Doris Del Zio given false hope when she was offered IVF as a solution to her infertility? Why did she believe her eggs could be successfully cultured and transferred to her uterus? Doris willingly submitted to a lengthy and painful operation and spent thousands of dollars on medical bills and travel expenses. She fought a long, drawn-out court battle because she thought her embryo had a good chance of survival. Why? Was it only her hope and desperation that fostered this belief, or was it also because IVF was presented to her by Sweeney and Shettles as a "possible therapeutic option"?

If Doris was in fact experimentally exploited, which man acted properly: Vande Wiele, who stopped the experiment because he believed it constituted unsafe and unethical human experimentation on human lives? Or Shettles, who was willing to go ahead with IVF and embryo transfer (ET) to please the Del Zios regardless of the experiment's effects on both mother and child? Since IVF hadn't yet been analyzed in higher mammals, why did Shettles consider it safe to try with humans? Why was Mrs. Del Zio given the impression her embryo might grow in her womb even though international researchers were years away from the first viable embryo transfer? It wasn't until 1981 that the first cattle were conceived by IVF and grew successfully in a cow's uterus.[11] Elizabeth Carr, America's first test-tube baby, arrived the same year. This is a staggering fact. One can't help but wonder: Do scientists think sex in a dish means the same thing to women as it does to cows? After all, IVF is a breeding technique, not a medical therapy. A woman who uses it isn't "cured" of anything—she is "made pregnant" by a team of IVF technicians.

In 1971, two years before the Del Zio tragedy, a physician at the National Research Council clearly foresaw the dilemma that would eventually be imposed on infertile women and society as a result of advanced reproductive technologies. In an article appearing in the *New England Journal of Medicine*, bioethicist Dr. Leon Kass cautioned:

> To consider infertility solely in terms of the traditional medical model of disease (or in terms of a so-called right of an individual to have a child) can only help to undermine, both in thought and in practice, the bond between childbearing and the covenant of marriage. In a technological age, viewing infertility as a disease demanding treatment by physicians fosters the development and encourages the use of all the new technologies [superovulation, egg harvesting, IVF, laboratory testing of embryos, and embryo transfer].
>
> Just as infertility is not a disease, so providing a child by artificial means to a woman with blocked oviducts is not treatment (as surgical reconstruction of her oviducts would be). She remains as infertile as before. What is being "treated" is her desire—a perfectly normal and unobjectionable desire—to bear a child. There is no clear medical therapeutic purpose that requires or demands the use of the new and untested technologies for initiating human life and that might possibly justify the unconsented-to use of a human subject [the mother and/or embryo] for the benefit of others and at risk to [her or] himself. . . .
>
> It is altogether too easy to exploit, even unwittingly, the desire of a childless couple. It would be cruel to generate for them false hopes (e.g., by exaggerated publicity). It would be

both cruel and unethical to generate hope falsely (e.g., by telling women that they themselves, rather than future infertile women, might be helped to have a child) to obtain their participation in experiments.[12]

What Do I Tell My Patients?

In Oldham, England, long before Doris Del Zio had ever heard of the term *in vitro fertilization,* dozens of other infertile women had also been told they had one last chance of bearing a child. Women with blocked tubes. Women who had tried every possible means to overcome their infertility. Women willing to endure repeated trials of ovarian stimulation and reproductive surgery in the hope of producing a baby.

After Robert Edwards and Barry Bavister successfully fertilized those twelve human eggs in a petri dish at Cambridge University, the next question was how to get embryos to grow following the procedure. In order to accomplish this, Edwards knew he would have a better chance of success if he obtained mature eggs. Up until then, he had ripened ova in culture fluid using eggs swiped from women during gynecological surgery.

By joining forces with ob/gyn Patrick Steptoe, Edwards gained access to living ovaries at precisely the right moment of the menstrual cycle. Of this, Edwards says:

> It was a question then of Patrick obtaining the ripened eggs directly from women by laparoscopy—to withdraw eggs from the ovary without damaging them in any way. No one had ever done that before. But already I had evidence of Patrick's extraordinary surgical skill and his ability to use the laparoscope superbly.
>
> "Yes," said Patrick. "If we can find a way to aspirate [suction out] the eggs, laparoscopy should be invaluable for this purpose. It makes few demands on the patient, permits many manipulations in the abdominal cavity, and can be used repeatedly in the same patient."[13]

Before long Edwards and his research associate Jean Purdy invented an apparatus to be used during Steptoe's laparoscopies.

Basically its design allowed eggs to be vacuumed directly from mature ovarian follicles. Prior to surgery, volunteer subjects were given high doses of hormones to control their menstrual cycles and stimulate the ripening of the eggs—just as Edwards had done in mice a decade earlier. Then at what he hoped would be the perfect time, laparoscopies were performed to collect the eggs and begin culturing them in glass dishes. Unlike in his earlier trials with IVF, Edwards obtained the semen of patients' husbands to fertilize the eggs removed from Steptoe's patients.

In a limited way, the women operated upon were aware of Edwards's research. "We had to ask Patrick's infertile patients, those desperate for help and willing to undergo many trials in the hope of one day having their own babies, to cooperate in a project that was still in its stumbling early stages," he writes. "We soon discovered that patients needed to be restrained from volunteering too much. Patients would offer themselves for a second laparoscopy or even come to Oldham General Hospital twelve times a year if necessary!"[14]

On March 3, 1970, the *Washington Post* carried an announcement about the research. Of particular interest is the statement made by the woman from whom an egg was taken:

> Dr. Patrick Steptoe, who heads the team of doctors working on the [IVF] experiment, disclosed on television that he had extracted an ovum from a thirty-four-year-old housewife and fertilized it with her husband's sperm. The woman, Mrs. Sylvia Allen . . . said she hoped the fertilized ovum would be implanted in her womb in the next two to six weeks, meaning that the world's first baby conceived in a test tube could be born by the end of 1970.[15]

Mrs. Allen's embryo was never placed inside her body. The first embryo transfer at Oldham General Hospital did not take place until just before Christmas in 1971.[16]

Needless to say, Edwards finally had plenty of eggs and embryos to study. Human ova, once fertilized, were tested for growth in different culture mediums, including the reproductive tracts of rabbits:

The rabbit enjoyed the reputation of being a good embryo to grow, and also of being a good mother to support the embryos of other species; cow and sheep eggs will grow happily within the rabbit, and can even be flown around the world within it to establish herds in distant countries. We transferred some fertilized human eggs into rabbits to see if they would grow there, but they wouldn't.[17]

Environmental factors, such as incubation temperature, light exposure, and the chemicals used in culturing the embryos, were tested by observing embryos for their reactions to different substances. ("We had to test the fertilized human eggs in several different culture solutions to find which was best for their growth.")[18] Embryos that appeared to be growing normally were painstakingly examined for signs of damage or abnormality. Inspired by these experiments, Edwards writes:

> To observe a living, vibrant embryo beginning its earliest steps of development is a most stimulating sight for an embryologist, whether it be a mouse, rabbit, sea urchin, or human. . . .
> I am still thrilled as an egg divides and develops for, in addition to the beauty of its growth, the embryo is passing through a critical period of life of great exploration. It becomes magnificently organized, switching on its own biochemistry, increasing in size, and preparing itself quickly for implantation inside the womb. After that, its organs form—the cells gradually become capable of development into heart, lung, brain, eye. What a unique and wonderful process it is, as the increasing number of cells diverge and specialize in a delicate, integrated, and coordinated manner.[19]

One wonders: How can Robert Edwards justify walking where even angels fear to tread?

While Edwards was marveling at these events in the laboratory, infertile women were being told they had a chance at motherhood. They were experimentally injected with hormones, hospitalized, placed under general anesthesia, operated upon, and then sent home—without their embryos. Nine years of intensive research passed before the first embryo implanted successfully and survived until birth.

The first time the Steptoe and Edwards partnership produced several healthy-looking embryos, the event provoked an immediate confrontation. Steptoe, a physician, was confused about what his associate planned to do with the embryos and what to tell his patient if they were destroyed. For Edwards, an animal geneticist, there was no question about what must be done or how his partner should explain it:

> The temptation to replace the blastocysts [five-day-old embryos] into the mother on the spot was very strong, and I have often wondered what might have happened had we succumbed. They belonged not to us but to the wife and husband who had donated their eggs and spermatozoa.
>
> "What are we going to do with them?" asked Patrick.
>
> "We're going to flatten them for chromosomes," I replied.
>
> "What do I tell my patients?" Patrick insisted.
>
> Patrick knew, as I did, that there would always be some embryos that could not be replaced inside their mothers. Instead, they would have to be examined; they would have to be fixed and stained for microscopic examination, and, as a result, their growth ended. Was it justifiable to use these blastocysts so that we could investigate early human growth? Did they have any rights? . . . The embryos cleaving in our culture fluids were minute and immature without the vestige of an organ or even a tissue compared with those aborted under the law. . . .
>
> "What do I tell my patients?" Patrick had asked.
>
> "I've got to see that the cell nuclei and the chromosomes are good," I had replied. "You'll be able to explain to them that we've taken another step forward."[20]

Beginning with his first IVF success in October 1968,[21] it had been Edwards's practice to "flatten" the embryos he manufactured after observing them for signs of development. He did this in order to study their genetic makeup. "This was a heartbreaking procedure considering all the efforts we had made to obtain and nurture them,"

Edwards says. "But it had to be done to make sure they were growing normally."[22]

Until December 1971, Edwards claims he had no intention of returning these brand-new lives to their mothers.[23] The incident mentioned above occurred in 1969, more than two years before the first embryo was transferred to a woman's womb in Steptoe and Edwards's program.[24]

The first four embryos—and several dozen afterwards—were squashed, stained, and mounted on glass slides for examination. The question is, what did Patrick Steptoe tell his patients during those years? Why would women keep coming back to endure the experiments voluntarily if they believed there was no chance whatsoever of their offspring surviving in their wombs?

"Our patients were childless couples who hoped our research might enable them to have children," said Edwards of his subjects in 1970.[25] This, and nothing else, is what must have led the women to surrender their eggs to Cambridge's IVF technicians.

Outside the Law:
The Truth About Noncoital Reproduction Today

Surprisingly, IVF techniques, frequently portrayed by physicians to potential customers as "no longer experimental," had still not been accomplished in many mammals, including primates, before the techniques were tried on women.

In an article he wrote with his wife, Ruth Fowler, Robert Edwards admits to achieving human in vitro fertilization "with confirmatory observations on a few cow oocytes."[26] What exactly does this mean? Perhaps it means that the safety and efficacy of IVF was never proven by adequate trials in animals before being applied to humans. Doris Del Zio's story and Robert Edwards's experiments also demonstrate that IVF research took place without the fully informed and voluntary consent of the human subjects involved.[27]

Have researchers continued to exploit infertile couples as Leon Kass predicted? Are infertile women being adequately protected from unethical medical experimentation?

Consider that the widespread application of external fertilization procedures still takes place without the federal government's oversight and regulation of IVF's safety and effectiveness, of licensing requirements for practitioners, or of embryo laboratories. There are no governmental guidelines for training, uniform reporting of treatments and outcomes, standards for IVF/ET laboratory equipment, or recommendations for the use of advanced reproductive technologies.[28] Yet, amazingly, anyone who donates blood or submits a urine sample to any licensed medical facility in the United States is protected by all of these safeguards.

At a congressional hearing conducted by the Subcommittee on Regulation and Business Opportunities, IVF expert Dr. Richard Marrs was asked whether there were fewer regulations for embryo laboratories than for laboratories doing blood tests. Marrs replied:

> There are absolutely no regulations. The IVF [embryo] culture laboratories are not even a state recognized laboratory; they don't even exist in the minds of state regulatory agencies as far as licensing. We have to provide for our own hormonal laboratory in our center. We do our own hormonal measurement in blood and other plasma products; we have to give the state agency an updated monthly and quarterly analysis of our quality control, our variation of sampling, and we can be tested at any time by unknown samples that are sent from the state to be tested against our facility.
>
> Yet in the embryo laboratory we have made hundreds of babies from our embryo laboratory and it has yet to be put into any kind of quality control oversight. . . . when you see the number of clinics springing up from ten to almost two hundred in the last five years and the quality of outcome coming from over half of these clinics, I would have to say regulations need to take place because there is a lot of exploitation going on and I don't think the medical societies have the authority or power to do that. [Without government monitoring] I think we are going to self-destruct. I think with rampant use, and the uncontrolled use of these technologies, it would not be long before there would be major problems that would occur from the use of these technologies, and I think the public will then

lose faith in the ability of the physicians in this area to provide safe and optimistic treatment form.[29]

When Dr. Marrs presented guidelines on advanced reproductive technologies to members of the American Fertility Society, he said, "There was open hostility about requiring any type of reporting or credentialing." Discussion was tabled for a year, said Marrs, because "I was fearful of my life."[30]

In 1986 Marrs helped to found the Society for Assisted Reproductive Technology (SART), a credentialing process for IVF programs. Membership was open to IVF practitioners who conducted a minimum of forty treatment cycles yearly (in vitro fertilization cycles) and had a minimum of three live births. SART also demanded compliance with minimal standards for personnel and facilities as well as anonymous reporting of results to a central registry for annual publication. Even these minimum standards were met with "extreme hostility," said Marrs. Only 41 of the nation's IVF programs belonged to SART when it published its first report.[31]

IVF/ET research and related clinical programs proliferated rapidly during the fifteen years after the first IVF baby's birth in Great Britain (though more than half of the existing 170 American IVF clinics had not reported a single birth as of May 1988).[32] By 1993 the number of U.S. clinics offering IVF had climbed to 267. Additionally, IVF programs had been established in more than thirty-eight countries.[33] In 1994 the number of IVF births in the United States and Canada had reached 6,339.[34]

In an article titled "Easier Than Selling Soap," *Forbes* magazine estimates that in vitro programs represent a potential market worth over $460 million annually due to the rise in pelvic inflammatory disease and age-related infertility.[35] Citing additional evidence for this phenomenon, *Forbes* reports:

- One in every four IVF programs is operated on a for-profit basis and is owned by venture capitalists.
- IVF franchises have quickly proliferated from coast to coast.
- Where insurance coverage is mandated by state government, the high cost of IVF is no longer a barrier.

"Buffeted by the pressures of commercial interests and near-desperate patients searching for a technological miracle, the [IVF] technique has become a major player in an increasingly lucrative infertility market," notes a news report in the *Journal of the American Medical Association.* "In vitro fertilization has the potential to be a profit-making proposition because the pool of candidates is large."[36]

IVF/ET: A High-Tech, High-Risk, Low-Yield Business

In a rush to attract business, it has been common for IVF clinics to minimize the risks of the procedure to potential clients, quote success rates from other programs, and give confusing statistics that don't tell how many live births have resulted from ART.

"In the peculiar jargon of IVF/ET, 'success' is not a baby but a 'pregnancy.' And reported pregnancy rates are *not* pregnancies per number of women enrolled, nor women hormonally stimulated to superovulate, nor women from whom oocytes are retrieved," writes Madeleine H. Shearer, editor of *Birth.* "Women whose flesh does not pass these hurdles simply disappear from the clinics' statistics like ghosts."[37]

When doctors started asking one another to define pregnancy and questioned the efficacy of high-tech infertility treatments already in use, it was clear that something had gone quite wrong with the practice of medicine.[38] Even the top journals in reproductive medicine carried articles that raised serious doubts about the honesty and integrity of IVF practitioners.[39] Leading IVF technicians, recognizing their profession was not immune from unethical practices, wondered what to do about the growing crisis related to the commercialization of human reproduction.

"Some new IVF clinics seem more interested in selling stock than in actually serving customers," concludes the *Forbes* article. "Such facilities are mushrooming throughout the country . . . part of a burgeoning world of infertility specialists, research labs, and infertility drugs—all targeted at the growing number of infertile couples' quest for conception."[40]

Dr. Arthur Caplan, director of the Center for Biomedical Ethics at the University of Minnesota, describes the lengths to which some clinics will go to achieve "success":

> Fertility consumers are especially fragile customers. They are seeking any means to have a baby. They will go anywhere, spend any amount, to have a baby. They can be preyed upon. Centers often give average data. To me that is simply unethical in the area of informed consent.
>
> When one goes to a clinic, one does not care about pooled or averaged data. One wants to know what is the success rate in this clinic at this time. That must be provided, or informed consent is a charade. . . .
>
> IVF success rates are so discouraging that there are some centers trying to do better in terms of creating babies by using multiple [embryo] implants. It shows at the forty-one [leading] centers there were an average of three embryos used. Some centers use more than that. When they do, they sometimes create multiple pregnancies, three, four, five, or six babies.
>
> Then they use fetal reduction, which is killing some fetuses to preserve the health of the mother and to help the other fetuses survive. That is a serious procedure.[41]

It is incredible that physicians, going to such great lengths to produce babies by IVF, later intentionally destroy them in utero. Yet what Dr. Caplan is describing is now considered standard practice, an acceptable means of achieving "success" among an increasing number of infertility specialists.[42] By transplanting four to six embryos from the lab to the womb, the pregnancy rate significantly rises.[43]

In 1978 a leading British medical journal, *The Lancet*, carried the first published article on selective reduction of multiple pregnancy.[44] The paper describes a woman who voluntarily underwent amniocentesis for genetic diagnosis while carrying twins. Only one of her babies was found to have a genetically transmitted disorder. Both parents wished to avoid having the affected child and asked if the baby could be selectively aborted. The authors of the paper explain:

> During these discussions the possibility of trying to pierce the heart of the affected fetus was mentioned, but we emphasized

this procedure had not been done before and probably carried the risk of spontaneous abortion of the other fetus. After careful deliberation the parents decided to take this risk.[45]

The baby with Hurler's disease was aborted in the twenty-fourth week of pregnancy after two attempts to puncture the child's heart with a needle. The second twin was born nine weeks later by cesarean section. "Mother and child are in perfect health," concluded the physicians who performed the puncture. Yet they offered no follow-up study on the social and emotional effects of the selective abortion on the survivor or the family.[46]

In recent years this killing technique has gained popularity among some practitioners of reproductive medicine. The induction of multiple pregnancies in infertile women through the use of fertility drugs (gonadotropins) and IVF/ET are the primary factors underlying this development.[47] IVF technician Rene Frydman and his colleagues state:

> Ovarian stimulation for ovulation induction and in vitro fertilization (IVF) have increased the multiple pregnancy rate from less than 1 percent to about 20 percent. The pathology of multiple pregnancy is well documented and involves high perinatal morbidity and mortality associated with immaturity and prematurity.[48]

While claiming that the multiple pregnancy rate can be controlled "to some extent" by reducing the degree of ovarian stimulation or reducing the number of embryos transferred to the uterus, Frydman's team points out that multiple pregnancy will continue to remain the major complication related to fertility drugs and IVF/ET. Therefore, they conclude that "the development of a means by which the number of developing embryos can be controlled is of primary clinical importance."[49] Here is the description of the means they advocate:

> At ten week's gestation, a reduction in the number of embryos was performed at the Clamart Clinic in Paris. Guided by real-time ultrasonography and under abdominal

local anesthesia (lidocaine 1 percent), ten milliliters of amniotic fluid from each of the two sacs was aspirated [drawn out] through a ten centimeter long, 21 gauge needle. The tip of the needle was then directed into the thoracic [chest] cavity of the fetus and a mixture of 1 milliliter of dolosal and 3 milliliters of xylocaine was injected. The needle was left in place for up to ten minutes until cessation of cardiac activity was seen. If the initial injection was unsuccessful, it was repeated after ten minutes.[50]

Two babies were killed through the mother's abdomen via the lethal procedure. For at least twenty minutes, the woman had to lie with a needle piercing her womb as it slowly dispersed poison into her embryos' hearts. To recommend, let alone subject, a mother to this practice—especially after inducing the multiple pregnancy to begin with—is unconscionable.

Dr. Seymour Romney at the Albert Einstein College of Medicine in New York City suggests the term *selective reduction* be abandoned in favor of a "more positive" description. He recommends selective embryocide be called the "enhanced survival of multifetal pregnancies."[51]

Dr. Jerome Lejeune, the late French geneticist who discovered the chromosome for Down syndrome, was appropriately appalled by such descriptions of fetal destruction. "When medicine is used to reinforce natural selection," he says, "it is not any longer medicine; it is eugenics. It doesn't matter if the word is palatable or not; that is what it is."[52] (In addition to being one of the world's leading experts in human genetics, Lejeune was also a renowned advocate of persons with developmental disabilities and mental retardation.)

Stopping selective embryocide won't solve the primary problems associated with artificially induced conception. When the new technologies shift life-making from the heart of marriage to the realm of the laboratory, they do more than "assist" nature, they assault it. A third party—the IVF/ET technician—initiates and conducts the process instead of the mother's body. Consequently, eugenic diagnosis and embryo manipulation/experimentation become part and parcel of the in vitro reproductive process.[53] The entire context of reproduction is thus transformed by the ART technician. Instead of life spontaneously arising from the center of human sexuality, sperm and ova are mixed together in a glass petri dish under the selective scrutiny of scientists; the connection between intercourse and procreation is completely severed. In IVF/ET, a technique replaces the function and purpose of lovemaking—but at what price?

"What precisely is new about these new beginnings?" asks Dr. Leon Kass. Looking beyond the chronic sorrow of infertility, he eloquently reminds us to think about what it means to produce children in new ways:

> What is new is nothing more radical than the divorce of the generation of new human life from human sexuality and ultimately from the confines of the human body, a separation which began with artificial insemination and which will finish with ectogenesis, the full laboratory growth of a baby from sperm to term. What is new is that sexual intercourse will no longer be needed for generating new life. This novelty leads to two others: there is a new co-progenitor (or several such), the embryologist-geneticist-physician, and there is a new home for generation, the laboratory. The mysterious and intimate processes of generation are to be moved from the darkness of the womb to the bright (fluorescent) light of the laboratory, and beyond the shadow of a single doubt. . . .
>
> We are considering not merely new ways of beginning individual lives, but also—and this is far more important—new ways of life and new ways of viewing human life and the nature of man. A man is partly where he comes from, and the character of his life and his community will no doubt be influenced by (and will of course influence) the manner in which he comes to be.
>
> Human procreation not only issues in new human beings, it is itself a human activity (an activity of embodied men and women). . . . Moreover, the techniques that at first serve merely to provide a child to a childless couple will soon be used to exert control over the quality of the child. A new image of human procreation has been conceived, and a new "scientific" obstetrics will usher it into existence. As an obstetrician put it at a recent conference: "The business of obstetrics is to produce

optimum babies." The price to be paid for the optimum baby is the transfer of procreation from the home to the laboratory and its coincident transfer into manufacture.

Is there possibly some wisdom in the mystery of nature which joins the pleasure of sex, the communication of love, and the desire for children in the very activity by which we continue the chain of human existence?

To lay one's hands on human generation is to take a major step toward making man himself simply another of the man-made things.[54]

Women are not machines of reproduction, of course. We are each unique, individual persons in body, mind, and spirit. But ART technicians manipulate the biological aspects of maternity in spite of the tremendous physical, emotional, social, and spiritual costs associated with high-tech intervention in conception. In IVF the bond between intercourse and life is broken; life-making is displaced, disembodied, and disconnected from a woman's natural sexual experience; the joy of conception becomes a grueling battle against infertility in an expensive, painful procedure with a high failure rate. The fact is, making babies without making love is a high-risk, low-yield proposition for women and children.[55]

Doctors are willing to sell this service to women who voluntarily endure the ordeal in their quest for conception, just as Mrs. Del Zio did. But how many women fully understand the terms of the contract?

Chapter Three

The By-products of Manufactured Conception: Embryo Transplants

Although the proof of a baby—unlike that of a pudding—does not rest on its consumability, and in the case of man not even on its being born, efforts towards proving what is good for vegetables is also good for human beings are being continued in many places. The life of man is, however, an unrepeatable experiment: no controls, no placebos. Although the expectations facing, and also checking, a breeder of men must be much higher than those restraining the animal breeder, there will be no one around to do the reckoning and to settle the accounts when the time has come. Human husbandry is so new a profession that society has not yet learned how to protect itself.[1]

ERWIN CHARGAFF

Today industry-related protocols govern the storage of frozen semen and viable embryos. These precious "commodities" are then donated, sold, advertised, and traded.[2] As a result, a child may now be intentionally produced with the consent of five separate "parents": a *genetic mother* who produces the egg, a *genetic father* who provides the sperm, a *gestational mother* who carries the baby during pregnancy, and two *nurturing parents*—the adoptive mother and father—who will raise the child after she or he is born. But don't forget—if the *nurturing parents* get divorced and subsequently remarry, two more people—the *stepparents*—will be added to this mind-boggling scenario.

Think of it. Can you imagine what it would be like to be born into such a "family"? Barbara Katz Rothman, professor of sociology at the City University of New York, points out the implications:

Women never before were able to think about genetic motherhood without pregnancy, or pregnancy without genetic motherhood; if we were biological mothers (carrying babies), then
we were genetic mothers. But making the inseparable separate
is what the technology of reproduction is all about. And it is
this issue that we are now facing; women, for the first time,
have the potential for genetic parenthood without physiologic
motherhood. At all. No pregnancy. No birth. No suckling.
Women are about to become fathers.[3]

In the high-tech realm of laboratory reproduction, the wonder of
conception is desexualized, disembodied, and divorced from the
design of natural procreation. Consequently, the words *mother* and
father take on entirely new and different meanings.[4] Definitions of parenthood dissolve and are refashioned through experimental study and
barely tested scientific methods. Assorted couplings, tangled des-
tinies, and genetically disenfranchised offspring are the result.

"In the average situation, two parents with equal genetic investment in the child are unified by their mutual relationship to their
child," explains Ms. Sidney Callahan, professor of social psychology at Mercy College in New York. "They are irreversibly connected
and made kin through the biological child they have procreated."[5]
She adds:

With third-party or gestational donors, however, the exclusive
marital unity and equal biological bond is divided. One parent
will be related biologically to the child; the other parent will
not. True, the bypassed parent may have given consent, but
consent, even if truly informed and uncoerced, can hardly
equalize the imbalance. While there is certainly no real question of adultery in such a bypassing situation, nevertheless, the
intruding third-party donor, as in adultery, will inevitably be a
psychological reality in the couple's life. Even if there is no jeal-
ousy or envy, the reproductive inadequacy of one partner has
been reified and superceded by an outsider's potency, genetic
heritage, and superior reproductive capacity. Fertility and
reproduction have been given an overriding priority in the
couple's life. . . .

Fantasies about a child's past and future do make a difference, as all students of child development or family dynamics will attest. Third-party donors and surrogates cannot be counted on to disappear from family consciousness, even if legal contracts could control other ramifications or forbid actual interventions. . . .

It should be clear that adoption, which is a rescue of a child already in existence, is very different ethically from planning ahead of time to involve third-party donors in procuring a child. The adopted child, while perhaps harboring resentment against its birth parents, must look at its adopters differently from parents who have had him or her made to order. The "commodification of the child," drafting a child definitively into the service of parental will, is an infringement upon the child's dignity.[6]

Who Governs Medical Science?

The researchers who have made commercial reproduction possible say it isn't their job to investigate the human implications of their discoveries. If a given technique produces results, it is deemed acceptable—at least by a small minority of daring technicians bold enough to try it. Claiming that the ethical and spiritual questions are for philosophers and theologians, the work continues without consensus. Those who attempt to regulate new reproductive technologies are accused of placing "arbitrary limits" on valuable research. Scientists protect their turf by appointing likeminded ethicists to the groups that monitor their area of specialization. For example, the Board of Ethics of American Fertility Society (now called the American Society for Reproductive Medicine, or ASRM) has been primarily made up of practitioners of advanced infertility techniques.

"Medical ethics does not grow out of medical roots," bioethicist Dr. Leon Kass reminds us. "Therefore, medicine cannot be self-governing . . . the sciences of the workings of the body do not yield moral knowledge."[7]

The people, then, must govern medical science; it is up to us to decide what we will and will not allow. Princeton University professor Paul Ramsey believes that as a society, however, we have become more protective of our planetary environment than of our own species. In a two-part series written for the *Journal of the American Medical Association* he explains:

> While the leopard, the great whale, and the forests are to be protected by restoring in mankind a proper sense of things, man as a natural being is to be given no such protection. There are aspects of the cheetah's existence which ought not to be violated, but none of man's. Other species are to be protected in their natural habitat and in their natural functions, but man is not. . . .
>
> So today we have the oddity that men are preparing to play God over the human species while many among us are denying themselves that role over other species in nature. There is a renewed sense of the sacredness of groves, of the fact that the air and streams should not be violated. At the same time there is no abatement of acceptance of the view that human parenthood can be taken apart in Oxford, England, New York, and Washington, DC; and, of course, it follows that thereafter human nature has to be wrought by Predestinators in the Decanting and Conditioning Rooms of the East London Hatchery and in commercial firms bearing the name "Genetic Laboratories, Inc." in all our metropolitan centers.
>
> I have no explanation of why there is not among medical scientists an upsurge of protest against turning the profession of medical care into a technological function. . . . Still there seems to be an evident, simple explanation of why people generally in all the advanced industrial countries of the world are apt to raise no serious objection, or apt at least to yield, to what the manipulation of embryos will surely do to ourselves and our progeny. It is a final irony to realize why invasions will now be done on man that we are slowly learning not to do on other natural objects; why natural human "courses of action" will be disassembled in an age in which we have learned to deplore strip mining. In actual practice minerals and vegetables may be more respected than human parenthood, and mankind may be ushered happily into *Brave New World*.[8]

The reason for the acceptance of this new technology, Ramsey asserts, is because it is being accomplished by doctors, figures of authority whom we are taught to trust without question.

Is Ramsey's indictment of medicalized reproduction too extreme? If you find yourself doubting his analysis, then consider the sobering story of a company called Fertility and Genetics Research (FGR), Inc., founded in 1978.

Bargaining Over Babies

Founded by Richard G. Seed, a nuclear physicist turned biomedical engineer, and Dr. Randolph W. Seed, a surgeon, FGR was originally designed to become a for-profit chain of nationwide fertility clinics. Using a cattle-breeding technique they developed in the 1970s,[9] the Seeds' company offered embryo transplants through franchised medical clinics.[10]

The owners of Fertility and Genetics Research seemed to think that their network of independent technicians would eventually provide embryos to 30,000 to 50,000 women each year. In 1980 Richard Seed said the procedure would cost couples about "as much as a new car," adding, "It should be painful to them, otherwise it isn't worth our effort to work with them for a year or two."[11]

What price did FGR consider to be the going rate for human embryos? Seed estimated the final cost to be about $10,000 per child.[12] Others placed the price a little lower.

Obstetricians/gynecologists Dr. John E. Buster and Dr. Mark V. Sauer, who worked with Richard and Randolph Seed to develop the technique, concluded an article on the procedure with the following statement:

> During 1986, nonsurgical donor ovum transfer [i.e., embryo transplants] will become clinically available through a publicly held medical technology company (Fertility and Genetics Research, Inc., Chicago, IL). The first clinic will open in Los Angeles, and the company expects to open other centers throughout the United States shortly thereafter. The cost is expected to be approximately $6,000 to $7,000 for four donor

insemination attempts. [Additional information can be obtained by writing to: Fertility and Genetics Research, Inc., 624 South Grand Avenue, Suite 2900, Los Angeles, CA 90017.][13]

FGR Chairman Lawrence G. Sucsy, an investment banker, believed the business held the potential to make revenues of more than $50 million annually. Sucsy, who also owned a firm specializing in medical technology and computer-related companies, was intrigued by the idea when first approached by Richard Seed in 1977. It took nearly a year for him to commit to the project. He said that what finally persuaded him was a poll stating that 75 percent of the women surveyed approved of in vitro fertilization. "That convinced me that women would also accept embryo transfers," explained Sucsy.[14]

What exactly is the technique that FGR has promoted and sold? In short, it is a type of short-term surrogacy arrangement in which an artificially inseminated woman relinquishes her embryo after five to seven days of pregnancy. Another term for the procedure is *surrogate embryo transfer*, or SET.

In what is commonly known as "surrogate pregnancy," a woman is artificially inseminated with sperm from the husband of a woman unable to bear a child. If a pregnancy results, this woman—the baby's natural or "genetic" mother—carries the child until birth. She then gives her son or daughter to the child's father and his wife. However, surrogate motherhood isn't actually surrogacy in the true sense of the word. It's a third-party contract between the people who will raise the child—the baby's genetic father and the adoptive mother—and the genetic/gestational mother. The woman who carries the baby is not simply a "stand-in" for the adoptive mother; she is the child's actual mother, a woman who has chosen to give up her maternal rights according to the terms of a contractual agreement.

Embryo transplantation is surrogate motherhood with a twist. In this procedure, a woman is artificially inseminated with sperm from another woman's husband, but carries the embryo less than a week instead of waiting a full nine months to deliver the baby. The idea is for the woman—the "egg donor"—to conceive an embryo that can be flushed from her reproductive tract before it has a chance to implant in her uterus. Her embryo is then transferred to the womb of an adoptive mother to carry and give birth to the child.

Since it appears that any woman can carry another woman's baby, embryo flushing (or *uterine lavage*) and embryo transplantation make it possible for a wide variety of women to become pregnant. Women who are past menopause, who have no ovaries, who are carriers of a genetic disease, or whose tubes are impaired by disease or surgical sterilization are all possible candidates for this procedure.

Uterine lavage can also be used to transplant embryos into the wombs of women who wish to function as "gestational surrogates." In this procedure the flushed-out embryo is placed inside the womb of a woman who carries the baby during pregnancy, but gives the child to another woman after birth. The embryo comes from the genetic mother rather than the surrogate. Embryos produced by in vitro fertilization can be used this way as well.

As with other third-party pregnancy contracts, a pre-conception agreement requires the surrogate mother (who carries the baby) to relinquish the child at birth to the genetic father (from whose sperm the baby came) and his wife, the adoptive mother. However, if the baby was conceived using sperm provided by a donor, then both of the nurturing parents are adoptive parents. (Remember the five-parent scenario mentioned earlier? This is it.)[15]

"$50 a Flush with a $200 Bonus If We Recover a Fertilized Egg"

On April 14, 1977, Richard and Randolph Seed presented their idea for embryo transplantation at an international infertility conference.[16] But their research was completely based on their experience with cattle, not on humans. An abstract of their session printed in the American Fertility Society's professional journal, *Fertility and Sterility*, reads:

> Bovine embryo transplant is a technically and commercially viable proposition—we have transplanted from over 100

donors into over 300 recipients. On the most recent 11 consecutive fertile donors, an average of 10.4 viable eggs were actually transferred. The donor is superovulated with [hormones]. Commercial cattlemen purchase the services on a per-pregnancy basis as a means of rapidly multiplying the offspring of superior genetic material. The donor embryos are recovered at five to eight days of age by a transcervical (nonsurgical) flushing, using modified tissue culture medium. . . . Liquid nitrogen freezing and long-term storage with normal live calves (but low yield) have also been reported. . . . Application to humans of these experimental animal techniques (immunologic, genetic, hormonal, transcervical) is straightforward. No adverse effects are expected.

Technology outpaces ethics. There exists neither political law nor theological law governing any aspect of human embryo transplants. It is perhaps time.[17]

The panel consisted of the Seeds and a veterinarian named Donald Baker. The three cattle-breeding specialists listed their address as the Embryo Transplant Corporation, Elgin, Illinois.

A year later Richard and Randolph Seed, along with Lawrence Sucsy, opened the first Fertility and Genetics Research program in commercial office space located in Chicago's elite Water Tower Place. By locating the Reproduction and Fertility Clinic in a fashionable retail area rather than a university medical center or private hospital, they successfully avoided publicity concerning the controversial techniques they planned to use.

"Our reception by and large has been quite favorable, but we structured it in such a way that there wasn't much negative that could be said about it," explains Richard Seed.[18]

"We expected we'd have pickets. We planned for pickets," he says. "It didn't happen."[19]

By 1980 the Seeds had a dozen interested couples with corresponding donors lined up to try their procedure.[20] Expecting to use the same donors over and over again, Richard Seed said they would pay all those who weren't volunteers "$50 a flush, with a $200 bonus if we recover a fertilized egg."[21]

Only two unfertilized eggs and one embryo had been recovered after two years.[22] The procedure, they discovered, turned out to be much more difficult to perform on women than it had been with cows. Yet they offered the program not as an experimental procedure, but as a professional service.

"The interval which traditionally separates a scientific discovery and its application in everyday life has been progressively shortened. As soon as a discovery is made, a concrete application is sought," writes French sociologist Jacques Ellul in *The Technological Society*. "The scientist might act more prudently; he might even be afraid to launch his carefully calculated laboratory findings into the world. But how can he resist the pressure of facts? How can he resist the pressure of money? How is he to resist success, publicity, public acclaim? Or the general state of mind which makes technical application the last word? How is he to resist the desire to pursue his research?"[23]

With determination, Richard and Randolph Seed pursued additional avenues of testing their cattle-breeding techniques. Soon they began working with a team of infertility specialists led by Dr. John E. Buster, a professor of obstetrics and gynecology at the Harbor-UCLA Medical Center in Torrance, California. The team spent four years and went through over fifty catheter designs before finally succeeding with the technique of embryo transplantation in a human being.[24]

"The uterus is a leaky organ," explains Buster, in an article appearing in *Fortune* magazine. "And the problem was to design an instrument that could recover the [fertilized] egg without flushing it out the cervix or into a fallopian tube, where it could cause a tubal pregnancy."[25] Considering that nature never intended the uterus to have embryos flushed out of it, it is not surprising that Buster's team ran into a few problems.

In 1987 the U.S. Patent Office issued patent number 5,005,583 for the embryo transfer procedure even after the American Fertility Society Ethics Committee condemned the technique's patenting as unethical. With the catheter design solved, the team began to improve—slightly—on its previous 100 percent failure rate. Called *nonsurgical ovum transfer* instead of embryo transplantation, Buster's method consisted of five steps:

STEP 1: An infertile patient is matched with a fertile donor according to genetic characteristics and blood type. Ovulation dates between the two women are synchronized by matching their menstrual cycles or administering fertility drugs. This is so the womb of the recipient is at the same point of the menstrual cycle as that of the donor at the time of the transplant.

STEP 2: When the cycles of the two women become closely matched, the donor is artificially inseminated at the clinic with sperm from the infertile recipient's husband.

STEP 3: On the fifth day after insemination, a plastic tube called a catheter is inserted into the donor's uterus. The physician then attempts to flush out the embryo with lavage fluid. The flushes, or lavages, are scheduled to allow the fertilized egg time to pass through the fallopian tube toward the uterus. The flushing is repeated on the sixth or seventh day after insemination, if necessary.

STEP 4: If an embryo is captured by the catheter, it must be located under a microscope and recovered from the lavage fluid. The embryo, if found, is then checked for signs of normal development. With improvements in embryo freezing techniques, the embryo can be chemically treated and quick-frozen after retrieval. The embryo is then kept in cold storage until the recipient's womb is ready to receive the embryo. Or the embryo may also be adopted by a suitable couple at a later date.[26]

STEP 5: As in in vitro fertilization, if the embryo is judged to be suitable for transfer it is placed directly into the recipient's uterus via a plastic tube inserted through the vagina and cervix.[27]

Egg donors for the Harbor-UCLA research project were primarily located through newspaper ads that read "Help an Infertile Woman Have a Baby."[28] Of the 380 women who responded, 46 were initially selected as potential candidates for the procedure. Psychological screening was then administered by the team's psychologists.[29] They found that abnormal psychological traits were threefold to sixfold more common among prospective donors than would have been expected within the general population.[30] Many of the women suffered from low self-esteem, while nearly one-third of the candidates had a history of abusive and/or alcoholic parents or other childhood problems.[31]

When classified ads turned up very few acceptable donors, John Buster and Richard and Randolph Seed came up with new ideas for locating subjects. These included encouraging infertile couples to find their own donors from among friends and relatives, placing brochures in doctors' waiting rooms, setting up a system similar to a blood bank where every embryo recipient would be required to recruit one or two donors, and hiring a public relations firm to send out press releases with a telephone listing for women interested in providing or receiving embryos. (The last four digits of the phone number spelled B-A-B-Y.)[32]

The UCLA donors were paid $5 to $10 for blood samples, $50 for inseminations, and $50 for uterine lavage. The team eventually flushed an embryo out of one woman and placed it into the womb of another in March 1983, three years after the project began.[33] By July two pregnancies were reported in a medical journal.[34] Six months later, in January 1984, one of the pregnancies resulted in the birth of a baby boy by cesarean section.[35]

The Five-Day Pregnancy

Between July 30, 1982, and February 5, 1987, twenty-seven female subjects were inseminated 115 times in this experimental study at the Harbor-UCLA Medical Center.[36] The research was funded by Richard and Randolph Seed's company, Fertility and Genetics Research, Inc.

Prior to insemination, all donors, recipients, and their respective husbands were asked to sign consent forms. Donor women and their husbands agreed to abstain from sexual intercourse near the time of ovulation. Subjects also were required to chemically or surgically abort their baby if the embryo implanted in the uterus.[37]

"The donors simply have to agree to an abortion," said Michael Eberhard of Memorial Health Technologies about the procedure. "If they won't, if that would not be emotionally or ethically acceptable to them, then we've got to screen them out. They don't belong as part of the donor program."[38]

During the study, 265 uterine lavages were performed on the twenty-seven women. Eight of the donors experienced more than twelve flushes each; one experienced fifty-three lavages.[39] A total of forty-three embryos were flushed out of their mothers' wombs and recovered from lavage fluid after undergoing microscopic scanning.[40] Clearly, most of the embryos did not survive. The number of births that resulted from the experiment is conspicuously missing from the article summarizing this research.

One of the donors experienced two retained pregnancies while participating in the experiment.[41] One of her embryos was lost through miscarriage, the other deliberately destroyed by abortion.

Physicians who performed the research concluded that the incidence of retained pregnancy "may be further lessened through the use of short-term, high-dose oral contraceptives (morning-after pill) or progesterone antagonists (RU486) taken immediately after a lavage sequence."[42] In other words, pregnancies induced by this method were guaranteed to be aborted—by lavage, by an abortifacient drug, or by vacuum aspiration.

In a later related experiment, six women underwent seven cycles of insemination and twenty-eight lavages after being "superovulated" with fertility drugs. (This is similar to what Randolph and Richard Seed had reported doing to cattle.) Doctors administered the high-risk drugs to donors in an attempt to stimulate the women's ovaries to produce more embryos.[43]

In a subsequent journal article, the research team reported:

Embryos were recovered from three of the women between 96 and 144 hours after ovulation. However, no ova were recovered from the other three donors, two of whom were later noted to be pregnant. Retained pregnancies occurred despite postlavage administration of high-dose oral contraceptive pills, endometrial aspiration, and, in one case, RU486. None of the infertile women became pregnant as a result of the trial. The authors conclude that although superovulation may increase ovum production, without reliable contragestion (i.e.

abortifacients), such practice is unsafe for ovum donors undergoing uterine lavage.[44]

Since none of the infertile women became pregnant and both the women who retained embryos aborted, the abortion rate for this experiment was 100 percent: All five embryos conceived during the experiment perished. What is more, every donor endured treatments to ensure their embryos would not implant in their wombs. Still, menstrual extraction, high doses of hormones, and RU486 failed to abort the two "retained pregnancies."

An article appearing in an issue of *Contemporary OB/GYN* announced: "OT [ovum transfer/embryo transplantation] may be repeated as many times as required to produce a pregnancy, with what appear to be negligible cumulative risks."[45]

What kind of medicine is this? Who and what is being treated by procedures such as these? This is not the practice of a healing art, the tending of the sick, the ministration of a cure: It is medically induced, manufactured (e.g., handmade) pregnancy—initiated and ended by technicians and machines. Why are physicians practicing and endorsing these dehumanizing, high-risk procedures?

Paul Ramsey offers an excellent answer to this question. The public will buy what advanced reproductive technologies offer

> ... [because] the agents of these vast changes are authority figures in white coats promising the benefits of applied knowledge. That, in other areas, we have learned to doubt in some degree. The deeper reason is that the agents of these vast changes, defendable step by defendable step, are deemed by the public to be not researchers mainly but members of the healing profession, those who care for us, who tend the human condition. Before it is realized that the objective has ceased to be the treatment of a *medical* condition, it will be too late; and Huxley will have been proved true.[46]

Beginning in 1978, Fertility and Genetics Research promoted embryo transplantation as a viable solution to infertility and genetic diseases. Founded by cattle-breeding experts, the company's goal was to establish embryo transplant centers throughout the United States. Physicians may be the ones who have applied Richard and Randolph Seed's methods to women, but these techniques do not belong to the practice of medicine. This is human breeding.

By calling embryo transplants "ovum transfers" and women who are artificially inseminated and lavaged "egg donors," medical technicians have applied inaccurate words to obscure the meaning of their activities.

Testing the Products of Conception

Though Lawrence Sucsy, FGR's chairman and chief executive officer, predicted the technique developed by the Seeds would be a big money-maker, surrogate embryo transfer turned out to be a costly proposition. In 1987, after FGR's balance sheet showed a loss of $316,289, Mr. Sucsy announced that his company would drop further attempts to create embryo transfer centers. But his company's name, Fertility and Genetics Research, Inc., points to other future possibilities beyond infertility treatment—the eventual application of this technology to prenatal diagnosis. As *Fortune* magazine, in discussing the possible applications of Sucsy's venture (and others like it), stated:

> The technique could replace amniocentesis, the prenatal test for Down syndrome and some other diseases; an embryo removed from its mother's womb could be tested for as many as 2,000 diseases and safely returned to her.
> Beyond that, Sucsy estimates that about 40 percent of the women who are waiting for FGR embryo transplants want to avoid passing on genetically transferred diseases such as hemophilia and cystic fibrosis. Eventually, with the development of new gene-altering techniques, doctors could remove an embryo from a woman with such a disease, alter the defective chromosomes, and return the embryo to the mother.[47]

Physicians John E. Buster and Mark V. Sauer affirm the natural link between embryo transplantation techniques and applied genetics. Speaking with the authority of those who pioneered the proce-

dure, they say, "Although first introduced for ovum [embryo] donation, the catheter may ultimately be used as a diagnostic tool in both
infertility and genetics. Collection of preimplantation embryos allows
diagnosis and treatment before implantation."[48]

Robert Edwards, a leading embryo technician, has always advo-
cated examining the embryos from the perspective of a geneticist.
Throughout his published writings he extols the virtues of identifying the genetic makeup of embryos for the purpose of preimplantation diagnosis.

"There is a wealth of information to be gained on the exact incidence and type of chromosome disorders in early human embryos
conceived in various circumstances," claims Edwards.[49] During the
early stages of his work with Patrick Steptoe, he wrote:

> The procedures leading to replacement and implantation open
> the way to further work on human embryos in the laboratory.
> . . . The basic procedure of embryo transfer will probably be
> combined with the identification of the sex of the embryo.
> Sexing can now be done with complete accuracy in the rabbit.
> The eugenic reason for sexing is that many genetic disorders
> are sex-linked; hence they usually occur in males.
>
> . . . the opportunity to give the mother a healthy embryo
> seems fundamentally humane. Sex-linked defects are only one
> sort of problem that might be avoided by the procedure; chro-
> mosome examination may one day prevent the birth of indi-
> viduals with genetic anomalies such as mongolism. . . .
>
> Further developments that also depend on the growth of
> human embryos perhaps contain the most controversial issues.
> These developments involve not simply identifying sex or
> genetic defects, but rather modifying or adding to the embryo
> itself.[50]

As a featured speaker at the annual meeting of the American
Gynecological Society at Colorado Springs in 1973, Edwards declared:

> The purpose of [my] work is to gain information about human
> conception, to use this information for the alleviation of cer-
> tain forms of human infertility, and to obtain a deeper aware-

ness of the physiologic events important to the development of
new methods in contraception, human genetics, and other
aspects of reproduction.

. . . the availability of cleaving human embryos could also
lead to the identification of those carrying specific genetic
[mutations] and provide a preferable alternative to the current
methods of aborting fetuses with anomalies. The preimplantation embryo can tolerate a considerable degree of interference;
pieces of [embryonic tissue] have been removed from rabbit,
mouse, and sheep blastocysts, and many of these embryos
develop to term despite the loss of tissue. If human embryos are
to be examined in this way for specific enzyme deficiencies, the
number of cells available for analysis would have to be increased
by culture or fusing them with other cells, and the embryo
would have to be maintained by frozen storage until typing was
completed. This possibility may be distant but perhaps not as
far fetched as it may sound, especially since mouse blastocysts
have been stored frozen at almost absolute zero. . . .[51]

"To undertake in vitro fertilization without guarding as far as possible against the birth of a handicapped child is indefensible," says
Edwards. "The clinical application of in vitro fertilization in all its
forms demands research on embryos . . . the embryo produced in vitro
is not a life which demands the protection of the law."[52]

"Preimplantation diagnosis" of human embryos is now possible
through the use of specially designed and patented genetic markers
called DNA "probes." Made of a particular sequence of DNA bases, a
specifically labeled gene probe is inserted into a cell's genetic material
and will bind to an identical sequence, thus showing up a "match."
Probes can detect extra or missing chromosomes, including male
Y-chromosomes in embryos four to eight days old.[53]

"It certainly wouldn't be ethical to use the method to choose the
sex of a baby," says Dr. John West of the University of Edinburgh's IVF
team, who developed the test. "But we wouldn't prevent the technique
from being used that way."[54]

Gene probes are already being marketed and used to detect hereditary diseases and genetic disorders in human embryos in interna-

tional IVF and embryo transplant clinics.[55] Down syndrome, cystic fibrosis, hemophilia, and muscular dystrophy are among the currently identifiable conditions. The Human Genome Project's map of the entire genetic code in human beings will make it possible to determine from the very beginning of life whether someone has acquired a specific genetic condition, disease, predisposition, or abnormality.

British embryologist Anne McLaren, a long-time proponent of prenatal diagnosis, eugenic abortion, and embryo experimentation, asserts, "Every pregnant woman wants to produce a normal healthy baby." Consequently, she says, prenatal diagnosis is in demand these days:

> Many older women avail themselves of amniocentesis, a procedure in which clinicians examine some of the cells shed by the fetus into the amniotic fluid. In Denmark, where such screening is widely available, the incidence of [Down syndrome] among babies born to women over thirty-five has fallen threefold since the 1970s. . . .
>
> The termination of a wanted pregnancy, even in the first trimester after chorionic villus sampling, is distressing. It means that a woman who seeks to have a child has to go through the first two months of pregnancy (often the worst part) to no avail. . . .
>
> If it were possible to diagnose genetic or chromosomal defects during the interval between fertilization and implantation—so-called "preimplantation diagnosis"—women "at risk" of producing a fetus with a severe genetic disease would indeed be able to start a pregnancy "in the knowledge that it would not be affected." One way for clinicians to carry out such diagnoses at this early stage would be to use *in vitro* fertilization (IVF) and then check the pre-embryos before replacing them in a woman's uterus. . . .[56]

McLaren then explains how embryos can be biopsied (have cells removed) for diagnosis and then suggests "the development of the biopsied embryos could be halted, while the tests were underway, by freezing them in nitrogen. Then doctors could select the unaffected ones for replacement in the uterus."[57]

Biopsy of embryos "might be the preferred strategy," suggests McLaren, for fertile couples desiring diagnosis before their embryo implants.[58] She explains that this can be accomplished by either using in vitro fertilization or, preferably, uterine lavage. Claiming "the flushing procedure is no more stressful for the woman than an insertion of an IUD," McLaren points out that the women can return to the clinic a month after the removal of their embryos "for the replacement of those blastocysts (embryos) found to be unaffected by the gene in question."[59]

"John Buster and his colleagues at the University of California at Los Angeles have found that recovering blastocysts in this way and replacing them," says McLaren, "gives a good pregnancy rate."[60]

A Biologist's Vision

The clarion call for the application of reproductive technology to selective breeding and the modification of human embryos was sounded in 1959. During that year, a small but significant book titled *Can Man Be Modified?* was received with much enthusiasm. Written by a French biologist named Jean Rostand, the book likely directly influenced men such as Robert Edwards. In it, Rostand details the responsibility of embryologists around the world to direct the course of human evolution.

Praising the visionary book *Brave New World*, Rostand contemplates the application of Aldous Huxley's vision:

This vision of the future is based upon precise knowledge of the present. To be sure, we cannot, for the moment, cultivate human embryos in test tubes, but already we can keep the embryos of rats, mice, rabbits, or guinea pigs alive for several days outside the womb; and the culture of embryos has indeed made considerable progress since Aldous Huxley wrote his *Brave New World*. (Etienne Wolff has succeeded with chickens in cultivating most of the embryonic organs—bones, eyes, the syrinx, the sexual glands, etc.). . . .

An intermediary solution of the problem of pregnancy is, indeed, conceivable. Delivery could be stimulated artificially and the embryo placed in culture at the age of two or three months. In short, a woman would reproduce like a kangaroo. If ever partial or total "test-tube pregnancy" came to be applied to our species, various operations would become possible, resulting in a more or less profound modification of the human being in the course of formation. It would then be no more than a game for the "man-farming biologist" to change the subject's sex, the color of its eyes, the general proportions of body and limbs, and perhaps the facial features. . . .

Can we, then, not hope to modify a whole stock, not just human individuals, in order to create a race or species of human beings superior to the present day? Even though we do not know exactly what is responsible for the intellectual power of different individuals, and if we merely start from the very probable postulate that it depends in part on hereditary conditions, it would be logical to try to reinforce it by using the method of artificial selection. This is a classic method, constantly used with success in plants and domestic animals. Every time it is proposed to accentuate this or that characteristic in a living stock, we choose as sires and dams the individuals that display this characteristic in the most marked degree. . . . If it were possible to apply similar methods to our own species, we should have no difficulty in creating stocks of men who would be taller or shorter, stronger or weaker, handsomer or uglier, etc. When we come to intellectual qualities the thing is less certain, but is still extremely probable.[61]

In the four decades that have passed since Jean Rostand's treatise on human embryology was published, his words have quickly progressed from the realm of scientific fantasy to reality. Human embryos have been tested for growth in the wombs of rabbits—not kangaroos—and "test-tube" conception is practiced at hundreds of clinics around the world. Embryo transplant franchises not only exist, but are now conducting business; advertisements for DNA probes have appeared in *Nature* magazine with full-page announcements in bright decorator colors. It is time to begin letting our governing representatives know this is not what we want for the future of our society.

Early Landmark Events in Reproductive Technology

IN ANIMALS		IN HUMANS
Use of artificial insemination in dogs	1782	
	1799	Pregnancy reported from artificial insemination
Birth from embryo transplantation in rabbits	1890s	
Use of cryoprotectant to successfully fully freeze and thaw animal sperm	1949	
First calf born after embryo transplantation	1951	
Live calf born after insemination with frozen sperm	1952	
	1953	First reported pregnancy after insemination with frozen sperm
Live rabbit offspring produced from in vitro fertilization (IVF)	1959	
Live offspring from frozen mouse embryos	1972	
	1976	First commercial surrogate motherhood arrangement reported in the United States
Transplantation of ovaries from one female to another in cattle	1978	Baby born after IVF in United Kingdom
	1980	Baby born after IVF in Australia
Calf born after IVF	1981	Baby born after IVF in United States
Sexing of embryos in rabbits Cattle embryos split to produce identical twins	1982	
	1983	Embryo transfer after uterine lavage (embryo flushing)
	1984	Baby born in Australia from embryo that was frozen and thawed
	1985	Baby born after gamete intrafallopian transfer (GIFT)
		First gestational surrogate arrangement reported in the United States
	1986	Baby born in the United States from embryo that was frozen and thawed

SOURCE: Office of Technology Assessment, 1988

Chapter Four

Making the Inseparable Separate: Artificial Wombs

Apart from medical uses, there is the great convenience for the mother of not having to undergo pregnancy at all, of skipping the morning sickness, the heavy step, the kicking fetus, the labor pains. Of course, there will remain staunch old-fashioned types who consider this more a deprivation than a convenience. Many people feel it would require a thorough-going revolution in ethics and morals to make this whole idea acceptable. Yet sex as recreation as opposed to sex as procreation has long since gained popular acceptance. And how many women have ever turned down labor-saving devices? Who would have predicted that so many millions of women would be so eager to interfere with their natural cycle of ovulation by dosing themselves with birth-control pills every day?[1]

ALBERT ROSENFELD, *THE SECOND GENESIS: THE COMING CONTROL OF LIFE*

As a child, I remember seeing a movie in elementary school foretelling the wonders of twenty-first-century technology. What stands out in my mind most clearly is a section of the film on the weather. Hurricanes, tornadoes, drought, and thunderstorms would all eventually be controlled by chemicals someday, the narrator said. A cartoon depicted clouds appearing and disappearing at the flick of a switch.

Several months later, *Life* magazine published a four-part series titled "On the Frontiers of Medicine: Control of Life." What astonished me most about the articles was a colorful picture of a stainless steel womb containing a living human fetus.[2] The accompanying text read:

> Like something out of *Brave New World*, the tiny human fetus in the porthole window at right is being kept alive in an artifi-

cial womb. Separated from its mother as a result of a miscarriage when it was just ten weeks old, it is still connected, via the umbilical cord, to the placenta, and it floats in fluid just as it would if it were preceding a normal birth. But nothing else is the same. This womb-with-a-view is made of thick steel because the highly oxygenated saline solution it contains is held under very high pressure—200 pounds per square inch, the same pressure a diver would encounter 450 feet down. At this pressure oxygen is literally forced through the skin of the fetus. Getting oxygen this way is called cutaneous respiration. But respiration also requires exhaling—getting rid of the waste carbon dioxide gas—and so far, the experimenter, Dr. Robert Goodlin of the Stanford University School of Medicine, has found no way to force out the poisonous carbon dioxide. Thus the fetus can only survive . . . for no more than forty-eight hours. . . .[3]

The strange photograph met all my youthful expectations regarding future scientific achievement. If space colonies and man-made weather would someday be a reality, why not this?

Years later, after giving birth to my own children, I returned to the picture in *Life* with an entirely different perspective. My immediate gut-level reaction was: *That's some woman's baby slowly being poisoned inside a stainless steel tank! Did they tell the mother her baby had been born alive? Was her permission obtained to use this still-kicking, sucking, swallowing fetus as a guinea pig? Didn't women back in 1965 wonder what this experimentation would eventually lead to—or were most people enthralled, as I once was, with the expanding use of reproductive technology?*

If experiments on artificial placentation were this advanced in 1965, then what is happening now? Why is the public no longer being informed about this research? Are babies still being slowly suffocated in similar experiments today? Could this be one of the many ways aborted "fetal tissue" is being used?[4]

I stared for a long time at the photograph of the perfectly formed child floating silently in the colorless fluid. I noticed that the picture had been taken by Lennart Nilsson. His awe-inspiring book, *A Child*

Is Born, had always fascinated me. Now that I knew how many of the pictures were obtained, I could no longer look at the book without feeling queasy.

While hopes of controlling weather have fallen flat in recent years, efforts to perfect the artificial womb continue unabated. "In San Francisco, researchers think we're only ten or fifteen years away from growing babies outside the womb," *USA Today* reported in 1989.[5] If this prediction is accurate, the technology I first saw in *Life* magazine is nearing implementation. Or is already in use.

Artificial Placentation Today

On December 1, 1968, the *American Journal of Obstetrics and Gynecology* printed an unusual article for a journal devoted to women's reproductive care. In "Maintenance of Sheep Fetuses by an Extracorporeal Circuit for Periods Up to 24 Hours," three British researchers report using sheep fetuses to test an artificial placenta.[6] Also called an *artificial perfusion unit*, the paper describes the mechanical exchange of blood through the umbilical vessels of the lambs and various ways to improve outcomes of the technique.

Nearly a year later, a similar article appeared in *Science* magazine: "Artificial Placenta: Two Days of Total Extrauterine Support of the Isolated Premature Lamb Fetus."[7] This time the experiments had taken place at the National Heart Institute just outside Washington, D.C. Reporting from the Laboratory of Technical Development, the authors explain:

> During perfusion, the fetus rested quietly in the artificial amniotic bath. About once each hour it moved its head or legs spontaneously. It exhibited a strong sucking reflex as well as a withdrawal reflex when pinched. After fifty-five hours of perfusion, the fetus abruptly underwent cardiac arrest [heart failure] and stopped extracting oxygen from the umbilical arterial blood. . . . Fetuses in four of the eight experiments survived for periods exceeding twenty hours, and we now have two apparently normal long-term surviving lambs after four and ten hours of extrauterine support.[8]

An illustration of a fetal lamb lying in a basin of fluid—with a circular tube leading away from and back to its umbilicus—appears on the first page of the article. A circuit containing two "pressure transducers," a "membrane oxygenator," pump, and IV bottle dispensing

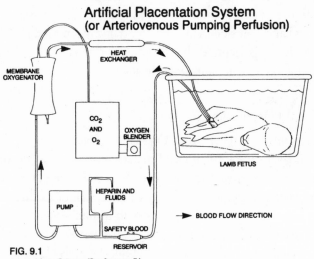

Artificial Placentation System
(or Arteriovenous Pumping Perfusion)

MEMBRANE OXYGENATOR

HEAT EXCHANGER

CO_2 AND O_2

OXYGEN BLENDER

LAMB FETUS

HEPARIN AND FLUIDS

PUMP

SAFETY BLOOD RESERVOIR

BLOOD FLOW DIRECTION

FIG. 9.1
Adapted from *Science*. (See footnote 7.)

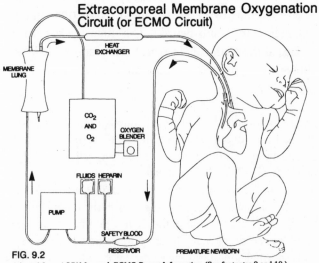

Extracorporeal Membrane Oxygenation
Circuit (or ECMO Circuit)

MEMBRANE LUNG

HEAT EXCHANGER

CO_2 AND O_2

OXYGEN BLENDER

FLUIDS HEPARIN

PUMP

SAFETY BLOOD RESERVOIR

PREMATURE NEWBORN

FIG. 9.2
Adapted from *AORN Journal, ECMO Parent Information*. (See footnotes 9 and 10.)

nutrients and a drug to prevent blood clotting make up the artificial placentation system (APS).

While I was writing the original edition of this book, a five-minute segment on a local news broadcast immediately caught my attention. I saw a human baby hooked up to a system *almost identical* to the one used for the lamb fetus. I knew it had to be the same device.

Afterwards I obtained a booklet describing the machine from the University of Nebraska Medical Center (UNMC), where the special news report had been taped. I wasn't surprised to see that it included an illustration that matched the one in *Science* magazine.[9] The drawings were dissimilar in only two respects. The human fetus was attached to the artificial placenta through the neck instead of at the umbilicus, and the synthetic amniotic fluid was missing.

Researchers who developed this unit apparently chose not to call it by its original name. It is now called an *extracorporeal membrane oxygenation (ECMO) unit*, rather than an artificial placentation system.[10] Is this to impress parents with high-tech terminology (difficult to pronounce and easy to abbreviate) or to deflect controversy?

Though early clinical trials began in 1975, ECMO has been in use around the country since 1980—primarily at university-affiliated neonatal intensive care units (NICUs).[11] ECMO, however, remains an expensive technology. Its cost is exorbitant, and it must be administered by highly trained personnel. Health-care providers maintain their skills by practicing the technique on sheep.

Robert T. Francoeur, professor of embryology at Farleigh-Dickinson University, tells of showing a film to teach students about artificial placentation in fetal lambs back in 1973. But he says "it was quickly withdrawn from circulation, and for about ten years no one heard anything definite about this research. People talked about the 'horrors' of an APS pregnancy, but with the film recalled and no one talking, there was no open 'enemy' on whom opposition could focus."[12] Evidently researchers have their reasons for staying quiet about this technology. But it is only a matter of time before society will be considered "ready" to accept mechanical gestation in some form.

Predicting that word of artificial placentation would resurface, Francoeur believed that the first artificial womb (from "sperm to term" as Leon Kass says) would be functioning by 1995. By that time, he apparently thought people would have adjusted "psychologically and emotionally" to the idea of mechanical motherhood.[13] Perhaps Francoeur assumed that after nearly twenty years of living with the reality of "test-tube babies," the artificial womb wouldn't seem strange anymore.

Yet 1995 came and went without any APS-related stories. This may be because, as with IVF and embryo transplants, APS is being introduced as a last-stop solution to a potentially lethal medical crisis. But history tells us that medical techniques have a way, in the course of time, of transforming the abnormal into the normal. The fact is, techniques are currently being used to produce human life extracorporeally (outside the body) and to maintain it extracorporeally at early gestational ages.

The womb is slowly being rendered nonessential to nurturing nascent life. Eventually it will be unnecessary for some women to conceive or carry a child inside their bodies. On the day that happens, biological motherhood will become technically obsolete.

Controlling Birth: The Ultimate Solution

In 1923 Margaret Sanger's book *Motherhood in Bondage* offered the following statements about the future of reproduction:

> In this era of standardization, during which most lives are planned externally if not autonomously, it is inevitable that the whole problem of rearing children will become as ordered, as controlled, as planned, as any other phase of life. Just as our finest fruits and flowers have been developed by choice and selection from wild flowers and wild trees, and our finest breeds of livestock have been developed by conscious control, so is humanity learning that the old traditional folkways, based on trial and error, have been too expensively tragic to the race at large.[14]

This current generation of American women is the first in history to collectively view the control of reproduction as a civic duty and personal right. To this end, millions have ingested mind-altering hormone drugs, used potent chemicals to create a "hostile vaginal environment" against live sperm, had their fallopian tubes surgically mutilated, had foreign objects implanted inside their wombs or arms, and—if all else failed or was accidentally forgotten—submitted to the destructive invasion of suction abortions. What is more, some physicians are now giving us the option to kill our *wanted* babies if they are the wrong sex, wrong genetic type, or wrong size.

Margaret Sanger, the founder of Planned Parenthood, was correct in predicting the eventual control of childbearing in a highly technological society. What Sanger didn't make clear, however, was that it would be women who would sacrifice their sexual integrity for standardized conception. Many have paid the price with their hearts as well as with their minds and bodies.

Curiously, men are not expected to alter the expression of their sexuality through invasive chemical treatments or killing. Women, not men, have been given the "choice" to repress and subvert their normal reproductive functions. Oral contraceptives, vaginal spermicides, tubal ligation, intrauterine devices, vacuum aspiration, and dilatation/evacuation have been sold to women as the medical means to "sexual liberation."

Rather than being freed to live in harmony with the natural rhythms of womanhood, women have been taught to fear what their wombs might produce—an unplanned pregnancy, a "defective" child, an untimely miscarriage. Some even say fertile women are "at-risk" of developing pregnancy—as if having a baby were a kind of cancer. But is it ever said that fertile men are "at-risk" of *producing* a pregnancy?

How many women in our nation are at peace with the natural state of their wombs, whether fertile or infertile? We are pressured from every direction to live in a continual state of denial and apprehension regarding our bodies' sexual capabilities and to use medicine to mask, bypass, or excise our nature.

"Pregnancy is the temporary deformation of the body of the individual for the sake of the species," according to feminist Shulamith Firestone. "Moreover childbirth *hurts*. And it isn't good for you."[15] In other words, the message here is: *Pregnancy is unhealthy, childbirth is abnormal, and normal reproductive behavior hurts women.* If even women come to view their bodies from such an anti-woman perspective, we can expect the practices of cesarean section, hysterectomy, abortion, and assisted reproductive technologies to continue flourishing in our culture.

"Artificial reproduction is not inherently dehumanizing," says Firestone. "At the very least, development of an option should make possible an honest reexamination of the ancient value of motherhood." She adds, "Until the taboo is lifted, until the decision to have children or not to have them 'naturally' is at least as legitimate as traditional [i.e., biological] childbearing, women are being forced into their female roles."[16]

Yet how can mechanical reproduction not be inherently dehumanizing? It is a strange type of "freedom" that would suggest women surrender pregnancy and the nurture of unborn children to machines. When this happens, children become the subject of scientific determination. Only the "best" and the "brightest" will be deemed worthy to survive.

The Man-Molders of the New Age

"One need only look at a tiny [human] fetus through the viewing porthole of Dr. Robert Goodlin's steel chamber at Stanford—or at a similar primate fetus, in this case still attached to its mother via the umbilical cord, at the University of Nevada—to see how convenient observation and treatment would be," explains Albert Rosenfeld. "Faults could be detected much more readily. . . ."[17]

As a woman, I find it incredible that members of my sex advocate the elimination of unborn children on the basis of gender or genetic quality. I associate this perspective of human life with militaristic-minded men and scientists motivated by utilitarian principles, not with mothers. Yet sex-selection abortions are already being done.[18] The ultimate solution to unwanted or "defective" children, once conceived, is to kill them.

If babies are already being killed following prenatal diagnosis—at as late as twenty-two weeks of pregnancy—what is going to happen when eight-celled embryos are found to be the wrong genetic type? When a four-week-old fetus floating in an artificial womb shows signs of physical deformation?

In *The Abolition of Man*, C. S. Lewis warns that "the man-molders of the new age will be armed with the powers of an omnicompetent state and an irresistible scientific technique: we shall get at last a race of conditioners who really can cut out all posterity in what shape they please."[19]

Make no mistake, children developing in a petri dish or an artificial womb will increasingly be judged according to their genetic value. Those found to be "substandard" will not pass quality control. Reproductive technology is a two-edged sword; its uses extend far beyond the treatment of infertility and infants born too early.

> At dinner he sat next to Filostrato. There were no other members of the inner circle within earshot. The Italian was in good spirits and talkative. He had just been given orders for the cutting down of some fine beech trees in the grounds.
>
> "Why have you done that, Professor?" said a Mr. Winter who sat opposite. "I shouldn't have thought they did much harm at that distance from the house. I'm rather fond of the trees myself."
>
> "Oh, yes, yes," replied Filostrato. "The pretty trees, the garden trees. But not the savages. I put the rose in the garden, but not the brier. The forest tree is a weed. But I tell you I have seen the civilized tree in Persia. It was a French attaché who had it because he was in a place where trees do not grow. It was made of metal. A poor, crude thing. But how if it were perfected? Light, made of aluminum. So natural, it would even deceive."
>
> "It would hardly be the same as a real tree," said Winter.
>
> "But consider the advantages! You get tired of him in one place; two workmen carry him somewhere else. It never dies. No leaves to fall, no twigs, no birds building nests, no muck and mess."
>
> "I suppose one or two, as curiosities, might be rather amusing."
>
> "Why one or two? At present, I allow, we must have forests, for the atmosphere. Presently we find a chemical substitute. And then, why any natural trees? I foresee nothing but the art tree all over the earth. In fact, we clean the planet."

"Do you mean," put in a man called Gould, "that we are to have no vegetation at all?"

"Exactly. You shave your face: even, in the English fashion, you shave him every day. One day we shave the planet."

"I wonder what the birds will make of it?"

"I would not have any birds either. On the art tree I would have the art birds all singing when you press a switch inside the house. When you are tired of the singing, you switch them off. Consider again the improvement. No feathers dropped about, no nests, no eggs, no dirt."

"It sounds," said Mark, "like abolishing pretty well all organic life."

"And why not? It is simple hygiene. Listen, my friends. If you pick up some rotten thing and find this organic life crawling over it, do you not say, 'Oh, the horrid thing. It is alive,' and then drop it?"

"Go on," said Winter.

"And you, especially you English, are you not hostile to any organic life except your own on your own body? Rather than permit it, you have invented the daily bath."

"That's true."

"And what do you call dirty dirt? Is it not precisely the organic? Minerals are clean dirt. But the real filth is what comes from organisms—sweat, spittle, excretions. Is not your whole idea of purity one huge example? The impure and the organic are interchangeable conceptions."

"What are you driving at, Professor?" said Gould. "After all, we are organisms ourselves."

"I grant it. That is the point. In us organic life has produced Mind. It has done its work. After that we want no more of it. We do not want the world any longer furred over with organic life, like what you call the blue mould—all sprouting and budding and breeding and decaying. We must get rid of it. By little and little, of course. Slowly we learn how. Learn to make our brains live with less and less body: learn to build our bodies directly with chemicals, no longer have to stuff them full of dead brutes and weeds. Learn how to reproduce ourselves without copulation."

"I don't think that would be much fun," said Winter.

"*My friend, you have already separated the Fun, as you call it, from fertility. The Fun itself begins to pass away. Bah! I know that is not what you think. But look at your English women. Six out of ten are frigid, are they not? You see? Nature herself begins to throw away the anachronism. When she has thrown it away, then real civilization becomes possible. You would understand if you were peasants. Who would try to work with stallions and bulls? No, no; we want geldings and oxen. There will never be peace and order and discipline so long as there is sex. When man has thrown it away, he will become finally governable.*"[20]

Chapter Five

To Catch a Falling Star: Infertility Diagnosis and Treatment

Many doctors and lay people think that the great technical advances in the past twenty years in treating infertility have led to high success rates in treatment, but this is a myth. Subspecialists often do not appreciate the limited therapeutic impact of the many diagnostic tests, and many couples achieve pregnancy independently of medical intervention.[1]

—DR. RICHARD J. LILFORD AND MAUREEN E. DALTON

> *Go, and catch a falling star,*
> *Get with child a mandrake root,*
> *Tell me, where all past years are,*
> *Or who cleft the Devil's foot.*

—JOHN DONNE

A proverb of Solomon portrays the yearning to bear a child as an unquenchable desire, comparing the barren womb to drought-stricken earth and raging fire (Proverbs 30:16). But until this century, folk remedies were the only possible solution medicine could offer.

Rachel's cry to her husband Jacob—"Give me children, or else I'll die!" (Genesis 30:1)—is expressed by women in a different way today. Rachel bargained for mandrake roots. Today medical technology is believed to possess the power to cure infertility.

The National Center for Health Statistics has estimated that approximately 2.1 million American couples are currently unable to conceive a child. They purchase a costly array of infertility treatments and services, including diagnostic tests and drug therapy, surrogacy arrangements, artificial insemination (AI), and newer assisted reproductive technologies (ARTs) such as in vitro fertilization and embryo transfer (IVF/ET), gamete intrafallopian transfer (GIFT), and surrogate embryo transfer (SET).

In the months following an infertility diagnosis, visits to physicians and clinics become a regular part of these couples' monthly schedule, turning testing, treatment, and the timing of intercourse into a way of life. Entering this unexplored territory can be disorienting and disheartening for couples, with no clearly marked road maps to follow.

Laying It Out on the Table

Convinced that modern treatments are highly effective, thousands of couples annually elect to endure the expense and risks of extensive "therapies." Understandably, they may believe that if they just try hard enough and long enough, something will finally work. This "hard enough/long enough" attitude often becomes a way of coping with the loss of control couples feel after an infertility diagnosis.

Treatments prescribed vary greatly in their effectiveness. What's more, determining the cause of infertility is difficult. For a large percentage of infertile couples—up to 20 percent—the cause remains unknown.[2] Even the results of various tests, such as semen analysis and the post-coital test, can show considerably different results when done at different times.

Since the diagnosis of infertility doesn't necessarily mean the inability to ever have children but rather difficulty in conceiving, the path leading to pregnancy can quickly become expensive and emotionally exhausting. Compounding this situation is the fact that medical and social choices facing infertile couples have escalated dramatically in recent years. Available options have created new problems as well as new opportunities. Most importantly, couples may have to decide when to stop trying every new treatment and whether to pursue high-tech or third-party solutions to achieving their primary goal—parenthood.

Although the procedures performed depend upon the situation of each particular couple, the following list describes the most common diagnostic measures used today:[3]

Infertility Tests and Treatments

Couple's history and physical exam: A complete health history may be the single most important diagnostic tool a physician can employ. It should include information on the couple's education, employment, personality, stimulant and substance use, medications and treatments, nutrition and diet, exercise, immunizations, surgical history, family health history, psychological history, and sexual history. The physical exam seeks possible physiological and anatomical causes of infertility.

Semen analysis: Basic characteristics of sperm and seminal fluid are examined, including the quantity and activity of the sperm.

Resting body temperature and other menstrual cycle mapping: Since the resting, or basal body temperature, changes during the menstrual cycle, charting these changes may help to pinpoint ovulation. The woman performs this procedure herself, so the cost involves only the price of the thermometer.

Cervical mucus evaluation: Another method of ovulation prediction relies upon examination of cervical mucus. Microscopic analysis of these secretions reveals hormone-related changes in the mucus.

Measurements of hormone levels: A patient's blood and urine are tested for levels of hormones related to ovulation.

Post-coital test: One to two days before ovulation, the couple has intercourse two to four hours before arriving at their physician's office; one to three samples of the deposited discharge is then taken from different areas along the length of the cervical canal and analyzed.

Infection screening: Tests for sexually transmitted diseases are included to determine whether reproductive loss may be associated with infection.

Sperm antibody test: Antibodies to sperm may be present in a woman's vaginal secretions; this test examines the sperm-mucus interaction.

Ultrasonography: High-frequency sound waves are used to obtain detailed outlines of the reproductive system, especially changes in the ovaries related to ovulation.

Endometrial biopsy: A hollow tube is passed through the cervix for removing a small amount of the uterine lining for microscopic examination. This is used to date the menstrual cycle.

Hysterosalpingogram: Radio-opaque dyes are slowly injected into the uterus while X-rays are taken to determine the condition of the fallopian tubes.

Laparoscopy: Doctor gains direct visualization of the female reproductive tract through an illuminated long, narrow instrument. Minor surgery can also be done during this procedure.

Hysteroscopy: Doctor gains direct visualization of the interior of the uterus through a long, narrow, illuminated instrument inserted through the cervix; also allows minor surgery to be conducted.

Hamster-egg penetration assay: The husband's sperm are incubated with hamster eggs, and the eggs are watched for signs of fertilization.

Different Kinds of Customers

Since 1968 the number of office visits to physicians for infertility-related services rose from about 600,000 to 1.6 million in 1984.[4] Estimates place the number of office visits in recent years at over two million annually. This quest leads many couples down a complex and emotionally rocky path where their hoped-for destination frequently remains out of reach.

Infertility specialists help to raise couples' expectations. "There is always another therapy that I can try and never a point at which I tell a husband and wife that they have done everything that there is to do," explains Dr. George Tagatz, director of the infertility clinic at the University of Minnesota Medical Center. "Even when we know the chances are slim, it's not up to us to tell someone when to quit."[5]

Dr. Wayne Decker, director of New York's Fertility Research Foundation, holds the same philosophy. One of his clients had 133 artificial inseminations and two operations before giving birth. "Should I have told her to stop trying?" Decker asks.[6]

On the other hand, couples like John and Joanne Smith of Maryland wish one of their three physicians had recommended quitting. Joanne has *endometriosis*. The tissue that lines the inside of the uterus begins growing outside the womb, often preventing the sperm from meeting the egg in the fallopian tubes. Joanne's situation was further complicated by cysts on her ovaries. She had four operations in five years in attempts to remove them.

"Each time, they'd take a piece of my ovary. So I was down to maybe half an ovary left," explains Joanne. At that point, a physician recommended in vitro fertilization—even though his clinic had never produced a baby by IVF. Because their insurance company refused to cover the $7,000 in vitro procedure, the Smiths turned down his proposal. "That's when we finally said, 'Enough's enough. Let's try the adoption route.'"

Infertile couples who can afford to pursue treatment may falsely assume that their physicians will tell them at what point they should stop trying. "There's no question that some couples are exploited," says Dr. Robert Rebar of Northwestern University School of Medicine. "But you have to ask, 'Are they intentionally exploited?' When the couple says they'll do anything to have a baby, it's very difficult for them to stop."[7] (Note: Most infertility specialists see it as their professional duty to offer all available and appropriate treatments to their clients. They are not neutral partners in a couple's medical treatment—they are paid providers who sell professional health-care services on a fee-per-service basis.)

Rebar and eleven other leading infertility specialists say "there are many forces driving the development of this problem":

- *The malpractice crisis*, which is forcing obstetricians into the subspecialty areas of gynecology without adequate training.
- *The development of new technologies*, which often occurs in an ethical and regulatory vacuum.
- *The entrance of for-profit organizations* into the infertility arena.[8]

William Winslade, professor of medical humanities at the University of Texas, comments on the potential for exploitation. "With infertile couples, we're dealing with different kinds of customers, people who are in stress and vulnerable and thus often spend too much money without thought," he asserts.[9] In his book *Choosing Life or Death*, Winslade and coauthor Judith Wilson Ross point out:

Infertility treatment, like much plastic surgery, is elective treatment, undergone at the patients' request to alter their lives but not, in any ordinary sense, to improve their health. As a result, despite the fact that most physicians who specialize in infertility treatment sincerely desire to help the couples who come to them, the field is ripe for commercialization. Economic interests may cross over and affect medical interests. Infertility physicians frequently use the word *desperate* to refer to their patients. An economically motivated physician faced with a desperate patient may go to extraordinary lengths to provide assistance.[10]

Former barriers to pregnancy—sterility, age, virginity, menopause, family status, infertility, and sexual preference—no longer necessarily limit a woman's ability to attempt conception. Given the menu of ARTs now available (see below), couples who choose to proceed cautiously run counter to the trend of plunging ahead with a we'll-try-anything approach.

The ARTs Menu

ART (Assisted Reproductive Technology): Any treatment, technique, or procedure that involves the manipulation of human eggs and/or sperm for the purpose of establishing a pregnancy.

Assisted Hatching: Scratching or scoring the outer covering of human eggs via micromanipulation of ova outside the woman's body to facilitate the embryonic growth process.

Embryo Freezing (cryopreservation): A technique for preserving developing human beings through freezing to allow embryos to be placed in storage until they are thawed at a later date for the purpose of transfer to a woman's womb. If the woman and man who donated their gametes (eggs and sperm) for laboratory fertilization decide they do not want to use or donate the embryo(s) to another couple, the embryos are either destroyed or used for ART experimentation by the couple's prearranged consent (given in writing before IVF is performed).

GIFT (Gamete Intrafallopian Transfer): The placement of sperm and harvested eggs into an unblocked fallopian tube through a laparoscope for fertilization inside the body. As a result, this ART does not involve any laboratory handling of human embryos.

ICSI (Intracytoplasmic Sperm Injection): The injection of a single sperm into a harvested human egg via micromanipulation (piercing the egg's outer covering with a specially prepared microscopic needle) for the purpose of fertilization.

Intrauterine insemination: Semen is placed directly into the uterus to bypass the vagina and cervix when vaginal abnormalities, cervical mucus deficiencies, and sperm motility problems exist.

IVF (In Vitro Fertilization): Conception occurring in laboratory apparatus following egg harvesting; the name literally means "in glass" fertilization.

Superovulation: Fertility drugs are given to induce multiple ovulation prior to insemination or egg harvesting.

SET (Surrogate Embryo Transfer): The transfer of an embryo from an IVF laboratory or from the womb of a fertile donor to the uterus of an infertile recipient who will attempt to carry the embryo to term.

Vaginal and/or cervical insemination: Semen is injected into the vagina or at the opening of the womb and left to swim up to the fallopian tubes.

ZIFT (Zygote Intrafallopian Transfer): A technique in which eggs are harvested from a woman's ovary and fertilized in the laboratory via IVF; the fertilized egg (zygote) is then placed inside a woman's fallopian tubes through a small abdominal incision.

Choices facing infertile couples have escalated dramatically in the last twenty years. There is no doubt that today's fertility drugs, techniques, and therapies have given hope to thousands of couples who would have been childless a generation ago. Until the 1960s, for example, women who had stopped ovulating simply stopped trying to become pregnant. Now two powerful drugs—known commercially as Clomid and Pergonal—have been used successfully by many of these women.

Fertility drugs carry certain costs, however. Clomid (clomiphene) costs between $4 and $8 per tablet in the United States, with a typical stimulation cycle requiring ten tablets of the drug. Pergonal (hMG),

Metrodin (FSH), and Fertinex (FSH) cost $50 or more per ampule.[11] In addition to being very expensive, these medications are associated with certain health risks, including:

- death
- ovarian cancer
- significantly increased rate of multiple pregnancy, associated with a higher risk of premature birth and neonatal mortality and morbidity
- increased incidence of ectopic pregnancy and breast cancer
- ovarian hyperstimulation syndrome, characterized by severe pelvic pain and ovarian enlargement, requiring hospitalization
- rupture of ovarian cysts and internal bleeding, which may require surgery to remove the affected ovarian tissue
- increased incidence of bloating, stomach and pelvic pain
- ovarian enlargement and formation of ovarian cysts
- blurred or double vision
- jaundice (yellowing of eyes and skin)
- shortness of breath caused by a thromboembolism
- nausea and vomiting
- abnormal uterine bleeding
- headaches, dizziness, lightheadedness
- nervousness and insomnia
- breast tenderness[12]

Clomiphene has been reported to cause vaginal tissue changes in mice undergoing prenatal development similar to those produced by DES (diethylstilbestrol).[13] What this will mean to the daughters of women who inadvertently were taking clomiphene during early pregnancy is not known.

Yet even the most effective drugs and treatments can only go so far in helping a couple to have a baby. American couples annually spend billions of dollars seeking pregnancy.[14] But how many couples fail to conceive a baby after spending tens of thousands of dollars trying?

According to a study by the United States Office of Technology Assessment, therapeutic success rates vary tremendously and as a whole remain disappointingly low. "As many as half of the infertile couples seeking treatment remain unsuccessful, despite trying various avenues of treatment," claims Dr. Gary Ellis, the study's director. "For as many as one in five couples, the cause is never found."[15]

Of the couples who do become pregnant, many conceive independently of their treatment. For the couples who will fail, how do they know when to stop?

Writer Katherine Bouton expresses the dilemma this way: "When you absolutely cannot have children, it's called sterility. When it seems to be taking an awfully long time but you still hope, it's called infertility. Infertility is worse."[16]

Eileen Aicardi, a pediatrician, and her husband, Dennis, spent four years enduring what she refers to as their "dehumanizing" bout with infertility tests and diagnosis. Making love according to a strict schedule and then "getting on a table and having sperm taken out of me" is one of the reasons why Eileen considers her experience dehumanizing.

She comments that her physician offered little comfort during this time. He once remarked: "All infertile women are depressed. See this box of Kleenex? I go through three boxes a day."

When Eileen's doctor gave her a prescription for medication that can cause low blood pressure and dizziness, she decided to seek a second opinion. Just after her new physician removed tissue that had been "acting like an IUD" inside her uterus, the doctor's office received a timely phone call: Would the obstetrician be willing to provide services to a pregnant teenager? The Aicardis made arrangements to adopt the baby. A few months later, Eileen became pregnant.

Since being diagnosed as infertile, Eileen has given birth to four children. The Aicardis received a double surprise in June of 1987. "After all those years of putting your bottom on a pillow for half an hour, to think I had twins!" she exclaims. "It proves it was totally out of control."[17]

Is There Actually an Infertility Crisis?

In spite of all the publicity about infertility, not everyone is convinced that the infertility rate is rising as rapidly as some say. In fact, the Office of Technology Assessment found that the overall incidence of infertility in the United States remained relatively *unchanged* between 1965 and 1982.[18]

Jane Menken, associate director of the Office of Population Research, and her colleagues at Princeton University point out that age-related infertility does not rise significantly until after a woman reaches thirty-five. "Fertility, compared with that of women twenty to twenty-four, is reduced on average by 6 percent for women twenty-five to twenty-nine, 14 percent for those thirty to thirty-four, and 31 percent for women thirty-five to thirty-nine, with much greater decline thereafter," they point out. Also their research indicates that women do not become infertile instantaneously. Instead, there is a period of declining ability to bear a child before sterility occurs.[19]

Under current medical practice, infertility is generally defined as "the inability of a couple to conceive after twelve months of intercourse without contraception."[20] Even for fertile women, however, Menken's group estimates that the mean time to conception is more than eight months and that at least 14 percent of those couples trying to have a baby take at least a year to conceive.[21]

This evidence is further supported by a two to seven-year follow-up study of 1,145 infertile couples published in the *New England Journal of Medicine*. In this group, 41 percent of the treated couples conceived, but so did 35 percent of the untreated couples.[22] Based on these findings, the researchers concluded:

- The spontaneous cure rate of infertility is high.
- Pregnancy occurs frequently in couples diagnosed as infertile but who have received no treatment or have stopped all treatment.
- For many infertile couples, the potential for conception without treatment is at least as high as with treatment.[23]

Do infertility specialists share this information with their clients? If not, why not?

"Clearly, the use of the one-year criterion as a measure of infertility confounds inability ever to conceive with difficulty in conceiving quickly," state Menken and her associates. "As a diagnostic tool, its advantage is that those with infertility problems have the opportunity to start treatment early. Nevertheless, because a substantial fraction of nonsterile couples takes more than a year to conceive, use of this criterion may generate needless anxiety in couples who hope to become parents and leads to unnecessary and costly medical treatment in a substantial proportion of cases."[24]

Other reasons for today's focus on infertility include:

Couples expect to be able to control fertility and plan parenthood according to schedule. After expending a great deal of effort turning off their reproductive ability, Americans think that controlling fertility is the main challenge, that getting pregnant is easy. It is hardly surprising, then, that many couples believe there are problems when a wanted child is not conceived quickly. Since there are fewer unintended pregnancies today, more couples are finally finding out how long it actually takes to achieve conception.

The birth rate is lower. With fewer women having fewer babies and more couples controlling fertility more effectively, not as many women need obstetrical services. Consequently, a larger proportion of women are coming to doctors' offices to have abortions or to obtain help with conception, not to get prenatal care. The situation appears even worse because many women are delaying childbearing.

The contraceptive revolution and the legalization of abortion, combined with the increased tendency for single mothers to raise their own babies, has drastically reduced the availability of adoptive children. Attention now focuses on the problems of disappointed couples instead.

Sexually transmitted infertility is on the rise. An overall increase in pelvic inflammatory disease, or PID, can lead to extensive scarring of the fallopian tubes. PID represents the greatest known threat—and also the most preventable danger—to women's fertility. The primary causes of PID are gonorrhea and chlamydia, sexually transmitted diseases that have reached epidemic levels during the past twenty years.[25] Such diseases account for an estimated 20 percent of all infertility in the United States.[26]

Intrauterine devices have also caused PID-related fertility loss in thousands of American women.[27] Up to 88,000 women have been estimated to be infertile due to using IUCDs as a birth control method.[28]

Temporary loss of fertility following use of oral contraceptives is common. Hormonal treatments may alleviate post-Pill infertility, but these involve diagnosis and expensive medication.[29] Oral contraceptive use also enhances the risk of infection with chlamydia, the leading cause of PID in the United States.[30]

Pelvic infections after abortion, surgery, or invasive diagnostic testing contribute to infertility by provoking tubal damage and scarring of reproductive tissue.

D&C (vacuum aspiration) during the late first trimester of pregnancy—and all abortions during the second trimester—pose a risk to women's fertility.[31] Therefore, increasing use of D&Cs and D&Es may be expected to contribute to infertility in the United States.

Smoking and drinking—habits practiced by many women of child-bearing age—have been linked to infertility.[32] Doctors in Boston studied more than 900 infertile women and found that smokers had more growths blocking their fallopian tubes and more changes in the cervical mucus that prevented sperm from reaching the uterus.[33] Compared to nonsmokers, women who smoke are three to four times more likely to take longer than one year to conceive.[34] Another study found that women who consumed more than one cup of coffee per day were half as likely to become pregnant, per cycle, as women who drank less.[35]

Other lifestyle factors related to infertility include regular strenuous exercise, poor nutrition, obesity, and stress. Women run an increased risk of reproductive impairment when repeated dieting, chronic stress, rapid weight loss, low body-fat levels, or excessive weight create hormonal imbalances.[36] All these factors are common among women today.

Infertility is over-diagnosed due to the medical definition of infertility. The standard one-year criterion has not been thoroughly researched; conflicting studies demonstrate that the length of time required for conception varies substantially from couple to couple. It is questionable whether the benefits of using so nonspecific a test outweigh the financial and emotional costs. Remember—for as many as one in five couples, the cause of infertility is never found.[37]

Excessive testing and diagnosis benefits our current health-care sys-

tem. Medical interventions for infertility generate business for doctors and hospitals. While physicians may provide infertility services partially out of compassion for their clients, their area of specialization also provides them with the challenge of mastering new skills and opportunities to boost their professional status.

New reproductive technologies—"test-tube" babies, surrogate mothers, surgical interventions for infertility, and reversal of sterilizing operations—have brought public attention to fertility problems, but have failed to adequately address causes of reproductive impairment. Also these expensive procedures are far from foolproof. Of the more than two billion dollars spent on infertility treatments and ARTs in the United States each year, a significant percentage goes to IVF clinics, with at least 45,000 couples using the techniques annually at $7,000-$13,000 per pregnancy attempt.[38] Yet the overall failure rate for IVF is still 85 to 90 percent.[39]

The picture of infertility being sold to the public is distorted by an overemphasis on treatment and too little focus on prevention. Infertility "is a problem requiring attention, but that attention should be directed toward disease and not distorted by an exaggerated impression of the effects of normal biological aging," concludes Menken's team. "The evidence indicates that the woman who deliberately postpones childbearing and either abstains from sex or participates in a monogamous relationship does not face great risks" of infertility.[40]

A letter appearing in the *Journal of the American Medical Association* sums up the issue well:

> Worldwide, approximately 5,000 children have been born as the result of (IVF). In the United States alone, there are about one million cases of pelvic inflammatory disease each year. If we assume that 130,000 to 500,000 of these cases lead to tubal occlusion [blockage], then in the United States alone *in one month or less*, pelvic inflammatory disease creates more new cases of infertility than have been successfully treated by all IVF programs in the world since Louise Brown was born in 1978.[41]

Why is so little attention being paid to infertility prevention and so much to in vitro fertilization? Why so little emphasis on the relationship between contraceptive methods and permanent reproductive impairment? To the role of monogamy in protecting women's reproductive competency?

Why are millions of dollars being spent on medical "miracle" treatments such as IVF when up to 50 percent of the infertility occurring in this country might be avoided through healthier lifestyles and earlier childbearing? When the effectiveness of infertility treatments have yet to be proven? When treatment-independent pregnancies are almost as common as pregnancies in women treated for infertility?

A New Kind of Medicine

Dr. Allen DeCherney, an infertility specialist at Yale-New Haven Hospital, believes that infertile couples suffer "a life crisis as devastating as any disease known to man" if they think they may be unable to become parents. He adds: "Telling a couple they can never have children is worse than telling a seventy-year-old he is dying of cancer."[42]

Compassionate physicians such as Dr. DeCherney are frequently quoted in popular magazine articles on infertility. But the commercialization of human reproduction has not been based on sympathy alone. With the declining birth rate, ob/gyns personally profit from the business infertile couples bring to their practices. "Normal" low-risk, nonsurgical obstetrics isn't especially lucrative these days when a one-hour diagnostic procedure such as a laparoscopy may yield nearly the same income as an OB package that includes ten to sixteen prenatal visits, the delivery itself, and a post-birth checkup.[43]

Consider this want ad appearing in the yellow pages of the *Wisconsin Medical Journal*:

> OB/GYN, board-certified or eligible, to join highly progressive, rapidly growing practice. Normal and high-risk obstetrics emphasized along with highest levels of infertility care (microsurgery, GIFT, IVF, Laparoscopic Laser Surgery) as well as extensive gynecology and surgery practice. Easy lake country or Milwaukee suburban living. Salary and guarantees to meet your needs with opportunity for partnership within one year. . . .[44]

To boost the business and expertise of infertility diagnosis and treatment, an entire subspecialty—*endocrinology/infertility*—has been created within the field of obstetrics and gynecology. Physicians who practice this specialty are called *reproductive endocrinologists.*

Endocrinology/infertility was not recognized as a certifiable subspecialty of obstetrics and gynecology until 1974. By 1978, 64 physicians had received board certification in this field; in 1982 the number had more than doubled to 135.[45] As of December 31, 1987, there were 287 board-certified reproductive endocrinologists of this type in the United States. The total had reached 758 by the end of 1999.[46]

This explosion in infertility specialization has fueled related research, which in turn has promoted the rampant development—and mass marketing—of new reproductive technologies. An article in the *Journal of the American Medical Association* offers the following insights on this phenomenon:

> From the mid-1960s to the mid-1970s, the number of births declined rapidly, creating a "baby bust" situation. During this interval, the annual number of births fell from more than four million per year to just above three million per year. Thus, medical specialists with a primary interest in women's health care [i.e., ob/gyns] were faced with a decreasing volume of patients requesting obstetric services. In part to fill this void, many obstetricians expanded their sphere of interest. . . .
>
> The increased physician interest in infertility problems, while initially stimulated by the technical improvements in diagnosis/treatment and the consultations of higher-income populations with infertility problems, itself stimulated further scientific research and patient consultations. Thus, the interactive process between health care providers and consumers, once set into motion, actually became an important factor reinforcing the growth and public visibility of the infertility field. . . .
>
> Recent advances in treating infertile couples have generated wide-spread publicity. The "test-tube babies" resulting from in vitro fertilization have raised hopes of barren couples that these advanced methods might be applicable to them. In addition, techniques and use of microsurgery have increased in recent years. Finally, the advantages of new drugs to enhance

fertility have also gained media attention. Continuously hit by press statements highlighting successes in treating infertility, infertile American couples have had their hopes raised of possibly overcoming their inability to conceive. Because of heightened expectations, an increasing proportion seek medical advice to correct their infertility.[47]

"Technology has given people unreasonably high expectations," says Shulamit Reinharz, a sociologist at Brandeis University. "Couples delay marriage and pregnancy, use contraceptives and stop, and then expect to conceive."[48]

The first generation with the ability to prevent the births they do not want, couples today have difficulty coping when they can't have the children they do want. Modern medicine induces infertility through oral contraceptives, vasectomy, and tubal ligation; it is also expected to undo infertility via techniques such as IVF, embryo transfer, and artificial insemination. When fertility is viewed as a controllable aspect of life, physicians are the primary mediators of the reproductive process. And the quality of the "product" produced by this process, a living human child, is increasingly subject to medical scrutiny and screening.

Chapter Six

When to Say STOP:
Questions and Concerns

---

*Each new power won by man is a power over men as well. Each advance
leaves him weaker as well as stronger.[1]*

C. S. LEWIS, THE ABOLITION OF MAN

This is the new era of eugenic consumerism.[2]

DR. ROGER GOSDEN, DESIGNING BABIES

M ost couples marry with the expectation that a child will come
into their lives as a result of their sexual union. When the time
seems right to start a family, they adjust their family-planning method
accordingly, duly noting the time of the next expected menstrual
period on the calendar. Because couples now have the ability to prevent the births they do not want, most assume they will conceive
quickly and easily once they start "trying" to have a baby. Susan and
Rod were typical newlyweds in this regard.[3]

"We had decided to wait about two years before starting our family," says Susan. "About eighteen months after we were married, I
went off the Pill so my system could get cleaned out before I became
pregnant.

"We were busy the next few years with church activities, several
moves, and numerous other things, so we were pleasantly surprised
when I found out I was pregnant," she continues. "Our joy quickly
turned to sadness when I miscarried at seven weeks. Some told me I'd
be pregnant again in no time (one of those thoughtless things people
say at difficult times.)"

But Susan didn't get pregnant again right away. "Not long afterwards, I began thinking that maybe there was something wrong, that

maybe there was a reason I wasn't getting pregnant as easily as my friends were," she remembers. "I managed to keep pushing these thoughts aside. My worries became a reality when our new pastor and his wife spoke of their years of pain in struggling with infertility. They voiced my own experience exactly—but *infertility* was such a scary sounding word."

Susan's story eventually ended happily: She conceived a child six months after starting on Clomid, an infertility drug that induces ovulation. Benjamin was born nearly eight years after Rod and Susan were married. Medical treatment, while costly and time-consuming, proved to be an effective remedy in their situation.

Tom and Susie share a different story about their search for parenthood.[4] After six years of marriage and fifteen months without using contraceptives, medical tests revealed that Tom would never be able to produce sperm.

"We were totally in shock," Susie explains. "We could not imagine why that would have happened to us. It was devastating to Tom."

In today's world of high-tech infertility treatment, however, Tom's diagnosis did not preclude a possible pregnancy for Susie. A physician could have performed artificial insemination using sperm from an anonymous "father" that may have enabled her to conceive and carry a baby of her own. A relatively inexpensive and easy-to-perform procedure, this technique—called AID (artificial insemination by donor) or DI (donor insemination)—is now used by at least 60,000 women each year in the United States. Though the inability to have children is often seen solely as the problem of women, studies have shown that men are the cause of couple infertility just as often as women, with up to 40 percent of cases due to male infertility problems, mostly due to low sperm count.[5]

After the diagnosis, Susie and Tom found themselves facing questions about whether or not to use AID. "Many of our friends wondered why we didn't try other methods of having children. Some suggested donor insemination, but we just didn't feel that was a natural way to have children," she points out. "It's not in keeping with God's design for procreation. I know a lot of people who have considered it, but we knew this wasn't the way God wanted us to have our family."

In coming to terms with the reality of their situation, Susie accepted the difficult diagnosis of her husband's involuntary sterility. "I truly thank God for providing me with an incredible amount of understanding," she says, "because *it didn't matter to me.* I had loved Tom for who he was, not because I thought he had sperm. I wanted to be understanding and didn't want him to blame himself."

Tom and Susie decided when to say "STOP" to medical treatment. The ready availability of AID was not reason enough for them to use it. Instead, they decided to enter the next phase of their life together as equal partners, and thus they chose adoption. They are now the parents of two children.

Debbie and Kevin decided to continue pursuing the medical route to pregnancy even after they had spent over $35,000 and ninety-two grueling months in treatment. "To not go through this," asserts Debbie, "would make me feel like it was my fault, because I wasn't willing to try. No one, not even I, can look at me today and say, 'If you really wanted a biological child, you could have one.'"[6]

Debbie offers the following description of the initial phase of her infertility treatment:

> I [took] my basal body temperature approximately 1,260 times for forty-five consecutive months. . . . And that is the easy part. During the diagnostic phase, I had three endometrial biopsies—which consists of taking tissue from the inside of the uterus to determine hormone levels—and two post-coital tests—removal of the cervical mucus [following intercourse] to analyze sperm activity. . . . I have also had two diagnostic laparoscopies—the navel surgery done with general anesthesia to look at the ovaries, tubes, and uterus. The second of these surgeries included a hysteroscopy—examination of the inside of the uterus—and a D&C. . . . All of that comprised the diagnostic workup. My diagnosis was unexplained infertility.[7]

Debbie has also endured three miscarriages, six months of artificial insemination, one year of hormonal treatment, several additional surgeries, in vitro fertilization, and many weeks of daily drug injections to stimulate ovulation. When last interviewed, she and her husband, Kevin, were attempting to achieve pregnancy via sperm washing.

Debbie explains:

> As you can see, this type of care requires a great deal of time off work, not to mention money. My husband is a D.C. Police Detective, and his federal insurance does not cover infertility. Luckily, I was able to extend my Maryland insurance on an individual basis, but not everything is covered. Most insurance companies don't cover these procedures.
>
> Considering the present state of medical technology and research in infertility, I will probably never have a biological child. I won't be able to produce a child who will have my husband's smile and his wonderful eyes. And that thought is devastating to me and my family.[8]

Babies at Any Cost

Each year infertile couples spend ever-increasing amounts of time, money, and energy on medical treatment and infertility services. These services, once a relatively obscure medical specialty, have become big business—a burgeoning multibillion-dollar-a-year medical industry with an estimated five million potential customers.[9] Many have already discovered that the possibilities appear to be almost endless—and how difficult it is to decide what treatments to use and when to use them.

Since the diagnosis of infertility does not necessarily mean the inability to ever have children but rather difficulty in conceiving, the complicated path leading to a hoped-for pregnancy can rapidly become expensive and exhausting. The appeal of new reproductive technologies to infertile couples is understandably irresistible. But it is doubtful that couples completely understand what is involved before electing to embark on their procreative journey.

Because reproductive technologies are evolving faster than our ability to form a consensus on limits, new ARTs are developed, researched, and implemented before social scrutiny guides or restricts a technique's application. Without moral or legal limits to use as a compass, new directions in infertility treatment are negotiated by health-care consumers—couples who are often willing to try anything presented to them. Ethical guidelines, where they do exist, are selected and voted upon by the same health-care providers who perform and profit from the ART procedures.

"While we don't have mandates, our position is that we offer *guidance* to our members," explains Joyce Zeitz, public relations coordinator for the organization formerly known as the American Fertility Society (AFS) in Birmingham, Alabama, now called the American Society for Reproductive Medicine. "We came out with our first ethics report back in 1986. We now have ethics committees working independently. [Later reports cover] such areas as the use of donated eggs for menopausal women and preimplantation genetic diagnosis." Concerning these techniques and other artificial conception methods such as embryo splitting, Zeitz says the ASRM's official position is that "research should continue in these areas."

In Europe legislative bodies are considering or have already implemented a wide range of restrictions. French officials have proposed prohibiting IVF in post-menopausal women; Italy has announced plans to limit artificial conception and cloning; commercial surrogacy and cloning have been outlawed in Great Britain. In West Germany, where memories of the Nazi experiments still trouble a new generation of scientists, embryo experimentation and fertilization by donors has been banned.

Until recently in the United States, federal funding for embryo research was withdrawn under the Reagan and Bush administrations. As testing was conducted with government monies elsewhere—primarily in Great Britain and France—studies remained privately funded here. In January 1993, two days after assuming the presidency, on the twentieth anniversary of the Supreme Court's *Roe v. Wade* decision, President Clinton lifted the previous restrictions. Federal legislators later saw the risks, however, and passed a ban on federal funding of fetal tissue research in 1995. The ban is currently under debate.

As to cloning, California and Rhode Island have enacted temporary bans while Michigan has permanently outlawed human cloning efforts. A number of other states are now considering bills banning human cloning. On a federal level, several versions of human cloning bans are pending in Congress. (Please contact your elected representatives for current information on this legislation and let them know your opinion.)

With current widely used prenatal diagnostic techniques such as chorionic villus sampling and amniocentesis, parents wait ten to fifteen weeks until discovering whether their baby has a genetic disability, with second trimester abortion offered as a "solution" to the child's health condition. Embryo diagnosis, as discussed in an earlier chapter, offers a much earlier alternative: After a woman's egg is fertilized in a petri dish and develops to the eight-cell stage three days later, one cell is removed for DNA testing. If a defective gene is found, the embryo is discarded rather than transferred to the mother's womb. The test adds about $2,000 per IVF cycle. At least 500 genetically linked traits, including gender, have already been identified for possible diagnosis using this technique.

When the New England Genetics Research Institute conducted a study of 200 parents to better determine their attitudes regarding genetic screening of unborn children, the center asked: "For which genetic reasons would you abort a fetus?" While 1 percent said they would abort a baby of the "wrong" sex and 6 percent claimed they would abort their child if prenatal tests showed a predisposition to Alzheimer's disease, a staggering 11 percent reported they would abort an otherwise healthy child if she or he would likely be obese.[10] Apparently, the criteria for targeting developing human beings for destruction before they are born is continually expanding—and an elite corps of geneticists and infertility specialists are among the vanguard leading the assault.

"You have to accept that you're doing an abortion when you use IVF, if you believe that life begins at conception. But I don't believe life begins at conception," says IVF specialist Dr. Geoffrey Sher, a founder of the Pacific Fertility Medical Center in San Francisco. "We're doing all these things already by amniocentesis, etc. It's nothing new—it's just better and earlier."

Not everyone agrees with Dr. Sher that such powerful knowledge is necessary or desirable. "I worry about the possibility of making a

child into a product we consume, about whether we are turning ourselves into products to be manipulated at our own whim," says Dr.
Paul Lewis, Assistant Professor of Religion at St. Olaf College in
Northfield, Minnesota. "We can select for certain traits or not, and the
possibility of making a child exactly in our image—whatever hair
color, eye color, and IQ we want. It seems to me that we're in many
ways a consumer society where everything becomes a product that has
to be hawked and sold to the consumer market."

In the most comprehensive moral analysis of ARTs to date, the
Vatican's "Instruction on Respect for Human Life and the Dignity of
Procreation" condemns all types of prenatal genetic screening for the
purpose of aborting genetically disabled embryos and fetuses. (See
Appendix A.) Released in 1987, the statement declares that research
using human embryos "constitutes a crime against their dignity as
human beings." The statement questions the morality of IVF as a practice that "has required innumerable fertilizations and destruction of
human embryos."

"The human being must be respected—as a person—from the
very first instant of his existence," the document affirms. "A diagnosis which shows the existence of a malformation or a hereditary illness
must not be the equivalent of a death sentence."

Thinking Through the Issues

Is in vitro fertilization (IVF) a morally acceptable choice for
Christians? And what about artificial insemination by donor (AID)?
Both technologies offer possible answers to infertile couples con-
fronting specific reproductive disabilities, such as male sterility or
blocked fallopian tubes. If a couple coping with this kind of diagnosis can't have children without using one of these techniques, would
it be wrong to use it?

While these techniques seem superficially appealing, it's essential
to take a closer look and review the issues before answering this question. The appeal of ARTs to infertile couples is understandable, but do
most health-care consumers really understand the moral concerns
associated with child-making medical procedures?

I would like to see signs out in front of every infertility clinic with a warning printed in bright, bold letters: PROCEED WITH CAUTION. Before trying either IVF or AID, it is essential to think with the head as well as follow the heart. A couple's intense desire to have a baby is powerfully and understandably real, but it may make them especially vulnerable to medical exploitation. For those who value the sanctity of human life, there are a number of troubling moral concerns to think through regarding IVF and AID before choosing either of these options.

IVF and AID: A Summary of Moral Concerns

POINTS TO CONSIDER: IN VITRO FERTILIZATION (IVF)

IVF is not possible without extensive embryo research.[11] It is essential to remember that the first successful laboratory conception took place at Cambridge University in England when Robert G. Edwards, a geneticist, and a colleague used their own sperm to create embryos from eggs taken from a woman's surgically removed ovaries—without the woman's consent. Edwards then spent the next nine years experimenting with human embryos, including testing them for growth in the reproductive tracts of rabbits, explaining, "Embryos were grown during the early investigations without any intention of replacing them in the uterus, so that a minimum standard of success compatible with the introduction of a clinical programme to cure infertility could be attained."[12]

Dr. Georgeanna Jones, Edwards's American colleague and the reproductive endocrinologist at Eastern Virginia Medical School responsible for the first "test-tube" baby's birth in the U.S., believes *Roe v. Wade* was a "fortuitous" decision that allowed IVF research to proceed. Human life in the lab is, by necessity, expendable.

"The scientific research necessary to establish IVF as a clinical process involved the creation of human embryos which were used for research purposes," acknowledges Australian geneticist Karen Dawson. "Often they were destroyed in the process of the research. Some proposals for future research also involve the destruction of human embryos. Is such research morally acceptable? If so, under what circumstances?"[13]

What Dr. Dawson appears to be asking is: How else can IVF technicians continue to develop and improve this procedure than to experiment on the offspring of infertile couples? After the embryos have been created by laboratory technicians, placed in frozen storage, and the "extras" are unwanted by their parents, some scientists vehemently argue that it is a waste to dispose of such valuable "research material."

"It is crucially important to realize that, both historically and at present, the aim of scientists, medical practitioners and those others involved in the technique of IVF, is, and always has been, the attainment of higher rates of human pregnancy (or the alleviation of infertility) as well as progress in scientific and medical knowledge," notes ethicist Dr. Teresa Iglesias. "Their *primary* aim has never been, and *is not* in current practice, to provide an opportunity for each generated embryo, i.e., for each newly conceived human being, to continue to live and follow its normal course of development. It is in the actual *aim* with which the technique started and continues to be practised that its basic moral deficiency lies."[14] She adds:

> It is clear that there are two fundamental and related assumptions underlying the current ethical guidelines and practice of IVF. The first assumption is that *the early human embryo does not enjoy full human status*; the second assumption is that *the value and interests of science override the value and interests of the newly conceived human being.* The ground on which these assumptions rest constitutes the central problem of the present medico-ethical debate, and it constitutes the area where there is a great need for a conscientious position, scientifically informed, with moral, philosophical and theological insight. . . .[15]
>
> There really cannot be an ideal case for in vitro fertilization. IVF is not a morally permissible mode of generation for those who are committed to cherishing and caring for every individual human being from conception to death; IVF is not a course open to those who want to give life and love to a child just "for his own sake" as a person deserves.[16]

IVF commercializes human reproduction.[17] As of 1997 more than 350 infertility clinics were in business in the United States; twice as many are unlicensed.[18] All are virtually unregulated. Many IVF clinics in the United States are owned by venture capital investors and operated on a for-profit basis. In states where IVF is paid for by health insurance companies due to legislative mandate, IVF clinics are more plentiful. Some IVF clinics have never had a live birth.

"What you've got here is a very combustible mix," explains Oregon congressman Ron Wyden, "essentially no regulation, large sums of money, constantly changing and improving technology, and vulnerable couples who want to have a baby more than anything else on earth."[19]

It has been estimated that only 10 to 14 percent of couples who enroll in IVF programs in the United States actually succeed in having a live birth.[20] At a typical IVF clinic, it is not unlikely that a couple will spend between $44,000 and $200,000 to achieve a single pregnancy. (On average, the cost incurred per live birth increases from $66,667 for the first cycle of IVF to $114,286 by the sixth cycle, according to one study of the general population of couples undergoing IVF.)[21] With the cost for each IVF attempt amounting to $7,000 to $10,000,[22] one cannot help but weep for the hundreds of thousands of women who have bravely endured the pain and expense of this grueling procedure in hopes of having a baby and yet did not give birth to a living child.

IVF is a hit-and-miss, exorbitantly expensive technology that clearly favors those who can afford to pay the price. Consequently, its high cost discriminates against infertile couples who do not have the money or insurance coverage to pay for it. Social equity decidedly does not apply at IVF clinics across the country, where 99 percent of the customers are white.[23] Surely ART techniques profit infertility clinics far more than they benefit the average infertile American.

IVF frequently involves preimplantation diagnosis and the disposal of unwanted human embryos.[24] Since new technologies can detect the sex and certain genetic conditions of three-day-old embryos at the eight-cell stage of development, advocates of IVF argue that preimplantation diagnosis avoids the "necessity" of later abortions and expands the option of gender choice. The idea that only some lives are worthy to be lived is in direct conflict with the belief that every human life is a gift from God.

The growing interest in preimplantation embryo screening represents a profitable expansion of IVF services beyond infertility medicine because it potentially applies to *all* prospective parents who are willing to use IVF as a means of microscopically inspecting their developing offspring's gender and genetic makeup. Among the clinics that have started preimplantation genetic screening of IVF embryos are the Howard and Georgeanna Jones Institute for Reproductive Medicine in Norfolk, Virginia, where a forty-member research team launched its embryo-screening team in 1994; the Genetics and IVF Institute, another Virginia-based program that has marked a number of disorders for diagnosis, including sickle-cell anemia and cystic fibrosis; and Chicago's Illinois Masonic Medical Center, which in 1990 sponsored the First International Conference on Preimplantation Genetics, a symposium attended by over 250 researchers from across the globe.

"As the techniques of preimplantation genetic screening evolve, they may represent the ultimate tool in the genetic diagnosis of the unborn," observes attorney Andrew Kimbrell. "However, the genetic screening of preimplantation embryos also brings up troubling concerns about the legal and moral status of embryos. Is there a limit to how many 'inferior embryos' we can discard, or how often? And for what reasons is it permissible to destroy embryos? Do they have to be afflicted with serious genetic diseases, or can they be discarded for reasons having little to do with disease, such as the fact that the embryos may be of the 'wrong' sex or genetically predisposed to obesity or low I.Q.?"[25]

None of these questions have been answered. As Kimbrell explains, "As with so many reprotech advances, the new embryo screening is totally unregulated. The absence of legal limits on embryo screening leaves the door open to the creation of a new body shop business designed to provide couples with the 'perfect baby.'"[26]

IVF poses potential health risks to women and children.[27] We do not yet know the long-term effects of the high doses of hormones women receive while undergoing IVF. Nor do we know the effect these hormones will have upon their offspring. In addition, developing ova and embryos receive multiple exposures of ultrasound, which has yet to be declared universally safe in humans by the American Institute of Ultrasound in Medicine. Embryos are created "by hand" under artificial light, in man-made media, and incubated in a non-human environment. Whether this will negatively affect the health of those so created is currently unknown.

In response to congressional hearings that raised consumer protection issues in the IVF industry, the National Institute for Child Health and Development (NICHD) signed a five-year contract to collect medical data on 13,000 women undergoing ART at nine U.S. infertility clinics. Results from the NICHD study may not be available for a decade or longer.

Besides serious risks linked to the high rate of multiple pregnancies associated with IVF (see below), researchers and consumer groups cite concerns about cancer, birth defects, and other long-term health questions related to ARTs.

"I have become very concerned that the fertility drugs of the 1980s and 1990s will become the next DES story," explains Lucinda Finley, an expert on reproductive health law at the State University of New York. "DES (a synthetic hormone whose effects appeared after the daughters of women who took it during pregnancy reached puberty) was supposedly going to help reduce miscarriages and make babies bigger and healthier. Now it is the drugs that help people get pregnant that are being greeted with such enthusiasm," says Finley. "Women are being pumped up about these [drugs] without really knowing the long-term effects. I get very sobered by how little the pharmaceutical industry learns from each of its disasters."[28]

IVF significantly increases the likelihood of multiple conception and directly promotes the practice of selective abortion. One in three IVF births produces multiple children, a result of physicians transferring two, three, four, or more embryos per IVF attempt in order to boost pregnancy rates.[29] Yet the dangers of multiple births in comparison to single births are well documented:[30]

- The perinatal mortality rate in multiple-gestation pregnancies remains 3 to 10 times that in singleton pregnancies.
- Sixteen percent of babies born in multiple births die within the first month after birth, compared to 3 percent of single-born babies.
- Fifty-three percent of twins and 92 percent of triplets are born prematurely; 8 percent of singletons are premature.
- Seventy-eight percent of multiples are recipients of neonatal intensive care services, while only 15 percent of single-born babies require such care.

During prenatal development, babies in a multiple pregnancy run a higher risk of lung development problems and cranial hemorrhaging. They also run a significantly higher risk of developing significant chronic medical problems after birth, including cerebral palsy, lung disorders, blindness, deafness, and learning disabilities. For the mother, a multiple pregnancy raises the risk of gestational diabetes, increased incidence of premature birth, low-birth-weight babies, high blood pressure, uterine bleeding, and potentially life-threatening blood clots. Bed rest and drugs to arrest premature labor are frequently required. And, in most cases, cesarean section is the medically mandated method of delivery.

Because multiple births are associated with significantly increased risk for a mother and her preborn children, many physicians will recommend selective abortion as a legitimate solution to this technologically induced problem.[31]

"To maximize pregnancy rates, it is our practice to transfer four to six embryos to women if they are amenable to 'selective reduction,'" explains Dr. Geoffrey Sher.[32]

He adds, "Because an embryo's chance of survival is about 10 percent with conventional IVF and only higher (perhaps double) in cases of third-party parenting, enough embryos must be transferred into the uterus to ensure the highest possible birthrate. . . . We believe that couples should be made aware, in an unbiased manner, of the option of selective termination of pregnancy in a pro-choice environment."[33] Claiming that this procedure enhances the survival of her remaining unborn children, however, does not change the fact that the technique is designed to deliberately target human life in the womb for destruction.

"Like the proverbial traveling salesman who impregnates the farmer's daughter, the infertility doctors who use technology to create super-pregnancies seem untroubled by their results," notes Lori. B. Andrews. "They offer another technology: the termination of some of the fetuses. The physician injects potassium chloride into the heart of one or more of them. Usually the other fetuses survive, although the chance exists that the entire pregnancy will be miscarried. Doctors avoid the term *abortion*. They call the procedure *selective reduction*."[34]

IVF creates "surplus" embryos who must eventually be destroyed or donated to research programs if they are not implanted in women's wombs. "IVF—the term now used to describe the entire process from egg and sperm collection to embryo placement in the uterus—was developed originally for the purpose of curing one type of infertility," notes Princeton professor and biotechnology expert Lee M. Silver. "But what IVF does inherently, as well, is provide access to the egg and embryo. And with this access, it becomes possible to observe and modify the embryo and its genetic material before a pregnancy is initiated."[35]

There are currently an estimated 150,000 unclaimed or unwanted frozen embryos in the United States, all manufactured via IVF. Privately funded researchers have been dissecting embryos and growing human stem cells in the laboratory for years, though the use of tax dollars for federally funded embryo experiments was made off-limits in December 1998 by concerned legislators. (This was partially due to the fact that stem cells can be taken from a variety of sources, including adult body tissue. Stem cells are the foundation cells that our bodies utilize to build tissue and organs.) Recent hearings may once again remove the restrictions on embryo tampering. As some scientists have discovered, this "viable human material," i.e., living human beings in the earliest stages of life, could be especially useful to them for:[36]

- creating new contraceptives
- improving IVF techniques
- studying human reproduction and infertility

- designing detection methods for genetic and congenital abnormalities
- developing gene therapy and "germ-line engineering"[37]
- implanting stem cells in individuals afflicted by paralysis and chronic conditions such as Parkinson's disease and ALS (Lou Gehrig's disease)

"IVF provides a unique opportunity for the study of human reproduction and early development, with far-ranging implications for the treatment of infertility and for other areas of research," explains Dr. Karen Dawson. "There are several major areas of research dependent on embryo experimentation in which our present knowledge of this field is being added to."[38] But as Stephen Hall has noted in the *New York Times*, "in order to obtain human embryonic stem cells . . . you must destroy a human embryo."[39] And therein lies the moral problem.

IVF technologies increasingly use anonymous donors to obtain results.[40] Adopted children often desire to meet their birth parents in order to better answer the question, "Who am I?" What will happen when children are told that they were conceived with computer-selected gametes in a dish or rinsed out of an anonymous donor mother's womb after she was artificially inseminated at the doctor's office and then, as embryos, were placed in an unknown surrogate gestational mother's uterus?

No one knows the answer to this question; we have no studies to tell us what genetic disenfranchisement will mean to these youth. When sperm, ova, and embryos become commodities in the medical marketplace, what does this mean to the child who was "bought" and "produced" from anonymous donors?

"Anonymous donors become breeders," explains John T. Noonan, a professor of law at the University of California, Berkeley. "Its acceptance brings us to the worlds of Huxley and Orwell in which the final trick is played on the champions of procreation as a private choice. . . ."[41]

POINTS TO CONSIDER: EXTRAMARITAL INSEMINATION (AID)

Extramarital insemination commercializes and dehumanizes the father's role in procreation. A number of sperm banks around the country make it their business to provide for the collection and sale of human semen. Almost half of all women involved in artificial insemination (AI) are inseminated with sperm from anonymous donors who receive an average payment of $50 per "donation." Paid sperm donors are often medical students.[42] Some students make hundreds of such donations, providing semen as often as two to three times per week over several years. Lori B. Andrews, a legal expert in reproductive technology issues, reports that "donors" are paid to masturbate in soundproof booths—with pornographic material readily available—for a set fee.[43]

Vials of frozen semen are shipped to physicians who perform artificial insemination in their private offices or clinics. In recent years "do-it-yourself," at-home AID has become an attractive alternative to women desiring to bear children "without a man."[44]

Extramarital insemination is largely practiced without legal limits or reasonable consumer protections. Though fourteen states have statutes covering sperm donations, few require little more than testing semen for HIV. No government agency or professional group knows how many sperm banks exist. Yet in the United States today, over 11,000 physicians provide AI to about 172,000 women annually. Live births result in approximately 38 percent of cases. Each year an estimated 65,000 babies are born after AI, with about 30,000 of these births from donor inseminations.[45] Other estimates regarding the annual number of AID births range between 25,000 and 100,000. In reality, the actual number of babies born through AID is completely unknown.

There are also no legal limits on the number of children that can be created with a single donor's sperm. In a survey of AID practitioners, 88 percent declined to place limits on how many times a sperm donor could be used.[46] At commercial sperm banks where set limits do exist, some allow as many as 125 per donor.

Donor insemination laws in thirty-two states have declared that the husband of the woman who gives birth due to AID is the child's legal father, but only seventeen of these states specifically say that the provider of the sperm is not the legal father. Only fifteen states require doctors to file reports on the AID procedures they perform. These laws allow the files to be opened for review when a good reason exists—for example, to obtain the biological father's medical history[47] or, as has already happened in at least one case, to stop a marriage between a man and a woman fathered by the same donor.

"A medical doctor I interviewed created thirty-three children while a medical resident at Georgetown," reports Lori. B. Andrews. "He has provided in his will that if any of the sperm bank babies come calling, they will be allowed to take only $1 from his estate. To prevent intermarriage, he now tells his children by his wife, 'Don't marry anyone from D.C.'"[48]

Extramarital insemination fosters the eugenic "enhancement" of human offspring. Semen is kept in frozen storage and anonymously advertised in computer sheets listing such things as the sperm vendor's height, weight, hair and eye color, frame size, ethnic background, occupation, and favorite hobbies.[49] Over 90 percent of AID providers will match donors on request with their clients on the basis of eye color, complexion, and height; a majority of doctors will also match specifications regarding the donor's and client's intelligence quotient, educational attainment, and religious preference.[50] One sperm bank, the Repository of Germinal Choice in Escondido, California, sells semen samples obtained from exceptional scientists and athletes only, including the semen of Nobel prize winners.[51]

Nearly a third of practitioners with over one hundred AID clients offer sex selection enhancement to their customers. Called "sperm separation," this technique significantly increases a woman's odds of conceiving a child of preferred gender.[52] Future technological interventions will subject sperm to much more detailed preconception genetic screening.

Extramarital insemination fractures family bonds.[53] "The ethical dormancy about DI and sperm sale is puzzling," notes attorney Andrew Kimbrell, "for unlike the donation of many other bodily substances and parts, donated sperm can create the irreplaceable—a child."[54] And since the sperm is disembodied from its anonymous source, any child conceived by this procedure is automatically cut off from his or her father. Essentially, only the maternal side of one's genetic tree remains. This situation can lead to later problems. An engaged couple in Israel discovered shortly before their wedding that they had the same father and could not marry. Both had been the product of artificial insemination by donor.

Lest one compare this too closely with adoption, consider the primary difference: Adoption is the rescue of a child from abortion or abandonment who has already been conceived. AID is a prearranged third-party pregnancy that consciously creates a child to satisfy the wishes of the mother and nurturing father. Adopting a child who already exists is an act of self-giving and compassion, whereas the prearranged splicing of genetic bonds to obtain reproductive fulfillment is child-tampering.

"Every human being has a right to their heritage," asserted one AID child while searching for her dad.[55] A study conducted by the U.S. Office of Technology Assessment (OTA) discovered that only 3 percent of AID practitioners talk about the technique's potential psychological effects with AID recipients, and just 1 percent reported discussing the possible emotional ramifications for the women's husbands or offspring.[56]

Sometimes it is the sperm donor who suffers emotionally and spiritually as he ponders the child he will never know or see. "Two psychiatrists I know specialize in treating sperm donors who later experience regret," states attorney Lori Andrews. "In Canada a group of sperm donors banded together to try to find out more about the children they created. Robert Owen, a medical professor at the University of California, San Francisco, wonders about the children he created in the 1960s as a sperm donor at Harvard. 'Were they happy? Were they loved? Were they successful?' he asks himself."[57]

Extramarital insemination often results in deception about one's origins. Very few children conceived by heterosexual married couples using AID are told the truth about who their dad really is. In one study 85 percent of couples said they had not and would not inform their children they were conceived through paid donated sperm.[58] Consequently, most children born as the result of AID are brought up believing that the nurturing father is also the biological father. One eighteen-year-old woman was told at her mother's graveside by the man she had always assumed was her father that she was the product of AID.[59]

Extramarital insemination splits the couple in two from the moment of conception.[60] Only one spouse—the mother—has a biological connection to their child. During the pregnancy, she carries another man's baby in her womb rather than her husband's baby. Even if her husband claims it doesn't matter, he will constantly be reminded of his own inability to conceive a child with his wife as her equal partner in procreation.

What Are the Moral Limits?

Beyond the questions surrounding how society defines "life worthy of life," other thorny topics crop up with ARTs:

In what ways do family bonds change when five "parents" (sperm donor, egg donor, birth mother, and nurturing parents) are involved in making and raising a baby?

What happens when people are told they were conceived with computer-selected gametes or rinsed out of a surrogate mother's womb?

How will ARTs' availability shape our grandchildren's views of marriage, sexuality, and procreation?

Where does one draw the line in designing a baby—sex, intellect, body shape, eye color?

What are the moral limits as we face future developments in reproductive medicine?

We have yet to collectively answer these questions. There are no long-term studies, no prior generation's experiences, to predict ARTs' outcomes. Perhaps Professor Lewis says it best: "The Christian tradition—the Christian's notion of what God's purposes are—would lend itself to caution in pursuing these technologies. It calls us to radically redefine what it means to flourish."

Chapter Seven

Present and Future Possibilities: Embryo Manipulation, Cloning, Stem Cell Research, and Beyond

O Chestnut-tree, great-rooted,
Are you the leaf, the blossom or the bole?
O body swayed to music, O brightening glance,
How can we know the dancer from the dance?[1]

—W. B. YEATS, "AMONG SCHOOL CHILDREN"

A few years ago, I went to a free outdoor concert. It wasn't any old concert. Van Cliburn was playing a Tchaikovsky concerto with the Philadelphia Orchestra—Eugene Ormandy was conducting. That kind of wonderful sound you get to hear live only a few times in one lifetime.

In front of me sat half a dozen teenagers. Eating popcorn. That kind of sound has been made pretty often in the history of the world. But not often with Eugene Ormandy conducting. They might as well have been listening to a player piano.

That event has become a metaphor for me of how we live in God's universe. With little wonder. Little respect. We might as well live in a human-made garbage dump for all we appreciate the beauty and wonder God has surrounded us with. We scarcely seem able to distinguish between the Rocky Mountains and a Formica kitchen.[2]

—JOHN ALEXANDER

This book was written as a testimony about what is happening to one of nature's greatest masterpieces—the beauty and wonder of human reproduction. Through its historical analysis of documented facts and presentation of key questions regarding the ever-expanding application of ARTs, this book seeks to stimulate discussion in the hopes of promoting change.

The practices described in *Without Moral Limits* constitute a trend within the field of medicine characterized by:

- Utilitarian manipulation of human life in its earliest stages.
- Reliance upon drugs and medical technology.
- Use of invasive techniques to redirect and control natural life processes related to human reproduction.
- Materialistic values that place self-interest above the needs of society.

The surrender of fertility and reproduction to medical technology, rather than improving women's health, has in fact resulted in an unprecedented level of reproductive incompetence in our culture. The very people who benefit most from this crisis are those who have a vested interest in selling medical treatments and procedures. The more expensive, extensive, and extreme the technology is, the greater the benefit to the practitioner. But this is not necessarily true for the woman being treated. Where treatments are physician-referred and physician-monitored at the client's expense, it is the client and not the physician who pays the physical, emotional, and economic price of the technique or procedure.

In addition, these technologies foster a disregard for the dignity of women and the value of early human life. This area of medicine may be more appropriately called *gynetech* and *reprogenetics*—new words for a new kind of medicine that does not treat or heal but seeks to redefine the terms of fertility and reproduction. Oral contraceptives, after all, do not treat anything—unless one considers fertility or pregnancy a disease. In vitro fertilization, surrogate embryo transfer, and artificial insemination do not heal infertility; they are simply animal-breeding techniques applied to human beings. Prenatal diagnosis and eugenic abortion of children with Down syndrome or spina bifida are neither preventative nor therapeutic, but are strategies used to kill humans judged unworthy of life. The philosophy of traditional medicine is not behind these practices.

Toward What Kind of Future?

The business of gynetech and reprogenetics can grow only if we feed it with fear and ignorance, surrendering our wombs and ovaries to techniques that can neither help nor heal. By identifying the new medicine for what it actually is, we can effectively resist and restrict its influence as we warn others of its dangers.

Citizens of Great Britain and Australia have been engaged in heated public discussion and have drafted legislation concerning reproductive technologies and embryo experimentation since 1985.[3] Commercial surrogacy and human cloning have been banned in England, though the government may introduce legislation to amend the cloning ban to permit scientific research on embryo cells, raising the possibility Britain could be the first country to specifically authorize cloning from humans.[4] West Germany has placed a strict ban on IVF-related embryo research and is considering a ban on human cloning.[5] There is every reason to believe that we can accomplish the same protection for women and children here in the United States if we make our opinions known. But there is no time to lose.

Reproductive medicine produces harm, not healing, when it counterfeits the natural processes of reproduction, assaults human life with destructive techniques, and then uses it as a means to an end. A review of current predictions gleaned from recent scientific books and articles underscores the critical need for our thoughtful understanding and immediate resistance to utilitarian medicine.

Looking Toward the Future: The Frontiers of Life

Fetal farming. Unwanted fetuses and extra embryos are increasingly being viewed as a supply source of stem cells and organs for medical treatment in much the same way that fetal brain tissue is being used to treat Parkinson's disease today. According to *Time* magazine, ethicists are now debating the morality of transplanting ovaries from aborted fetuses into aging women. *USA Today* reports that "the prospect of scientists creating babies from the eggs of aborted fetuses—children whose 'mothers' were never born" may be accomplished within three years in humans. (British scientists have already perfected the technique in animals.)

R. G. Edwards suggests: "To grow fetuses to later stages of growth when they take a recognizable human shape and then extract their organs would be an utterly repugnant concept," he says in *A Matter of Life*, "but to obtain cell colonies from minute embryos useful in medicine for the alleviation of certain human disorders—is that not a legitimate target to aim at?"

UCLA cryogenics expert Paul Segall advocates a head-to-toe approach using a body clone: Once the clone grew to an appropriate size by intravenous feeding and hormone injections and was placed in frozen storage, it could later serve as the equivalent of a brain-dead organ donor with the same genetic makeup as the person from whom it was derived, thereby avoiding the possibility of transplant rejections.

Already researchers at private companies are taking stem cells from "surplus" human embryos created by IVF. But the federal government did not provide taxpayer money for research into embryonic stem cells after a December 1998 congressional ban was placed on any research that destroys human embryos. Yet the National Institutes of Health (NIH) is attempting to circumvent the ban by claiming that stem cells are preembryos—and that therefore research is allowable. Recent NIH guidelines will allow researchers to use federal funds for some embryonic stem cell research as long as the science is conducted only on cells already derived by private companies. In this way, NIH-funded scientists do not actually kill the embryos. Women will also be permitted to directly donate their extra IVF offspring to government-funded research programs.

Artificial wombs. Italian researchers have kept a surgically removed uterus functioning for fifty hours and believe breakthroughs in organ preservation techniques will eventually allow machine-assisted uteris and implanted embryos to remain viable for much longer. With artificial placentation systems employing ECMO (extra-corporeal membrane oxygenation) currently in use, it's only a matter of time before babies might be medically grown from "sperm to term," making biological motherhood technically obsolete.

Cloning, embryo "splitting," and selective breeding. Tests on cows' fertilized eggs proved that sixteen-cell embryos can be divided into four equal groups, cultured for a few days, and then redivided to yield sixteen identical clusters—each of which will grow into a genetically identical cow. The first laboratory duplication of human embryos by American researchers Jerry Hall and Robert Stillman in 1993, in which seventeen embryos were split into forty-eight, provoked intense ethical debate, but so far, no governmental restrictions. "It's up to the ethicists and the medical community, with input from the general public, to decide what kind of guidelines will lead us in the future," Hall said on *Larry King Live.*

On February 23, 1997, the world was introduced to a six-month-old lamb named Dolly that was cloned from an *adult* donor's cell taken from the breast tissue of a mature sheep. It was a feat that even expert geneticists and embryologists had doubted could be accomplished—the reprogramming of an adult mammal cell so that it would grow into a completely separate animal identical to the one born before its genetic copy.

"The cloning of Dolly broke the technological barrier. There is no reason to expect that the technology couldn't be transferred to human cells," declares Dr. Lee M. Silver. "On the contrary, there is every reason to expect that it *can* be transferred. It requires only equipment and facilities that are already standard or easy to obtain by biomedical laboratories and free-standing in vitro fertilization clinics across the country and across the world. Although the protocol itself demands the services of highly trained and skilled personnel, there are thousands of people with such skill in the United States alone."[6]

Primate surrogacy and male pregnancy. Someday scientists may be able to medically manipulate men to carry babies via hormones or implant human embryos in primate surrogates for gestation. A British scientist, Dr. R. V. Short, has proposed the creation of chimeras—a genetically combined ape-human species—to create a subclass to perform hazardous labor. Sounds like science fiction, but some researchers are dead serious about pushing the boundaries of reproductive technology to the outer reaches of man's imagination.

Some Statements Worth Thinking About: Unfounded Fears or Learned Predictions?

"We are looking at the same problem we had with nuclear power. In 1945, we dropped two bombs on Hiroshima and Nagasaki, then spent the next 50 years arguing the ethics of it. We chased that horse down the street after the barn door was already locked," testified Dr. Bernard Nathanson in February 2000 before congressional staff. Dr. Nathanson, a co-founder of the National Abortion and Reproductive Rights Action League, is now a leading expert on the impact of gynetech on medicine and society. Here are additional excerpts from his recent public speech:[7]

> Assisted reproductive technology is one of the hottest areas in modern medicine today. The first baby born in this country as a result of in-vitro fertilization was in 1981. In 1997, the last year for which we have any figures, there were 24,000 babies born of in-vitro fertilization. . . .
>
> This brings up the question as to whether infertility is a disease. Is it a medical disease to not become pregnant? . . .
>
> There is a very large market in frozen embryos. There are about 50,000 embryos in various cryobanks across the country. What are we to do?
>
> Freezing can only preserve an embryo five or six years. Some entrepreneurs have the answer: Sell them. One enterprising reporter showed that if you go to Columbia University, you can tell them what kind of baby you want, matching your physique, your ethnic background and your educational background, and they will pick out a frozen embryo that perfectly matches what you want and sell it to you and implant the embryo in the womb of your wife or girlfriend for all of $2,750. . . .
>
> There is technology such as posthumous sperm removal. If a man dies and the widow wants to become pregnant, within a reasonable period of time, the urologist puts a needle into the testes, pulls out some sperm and fertilizes her egg. So the dead man is a new father, reversing all normal familial relationships and procedures. . . .

Cloning has gotten completely out of hand, and it's potentially dangerous. . . . Dolly, the lamb that was created in Aberdeen, Scotland, has shown signs in its cells of premature aging. Nobody knows why. The Japanese have now cloned a bull from a cloned bull. They are cloning clones until the land is full of cloned bulls. These bulls, by the way, are fertile. They have cloned a calf from the ear cells of an adult cow, which means you don't need to use reproductive cells anymore. You can take any cell in the body, even from the inside of the mouth, and clone. . . . The South Koreans have admitted they are cloning human beings, and they are continuing the practice. . . .

There's something known as genetic enhancement that is being carried out on a large scale. . . . For example, if you want a child to be in the NBA and 6 feet 10 inches tall, at the embryo stage you'd ask that extra genes be put in for tallness. Or if you wanted extra memory so that you forget nothing, you put in more memory genes at the embryo stage. . . . All sorts of human mapping has been carried out. The entire human genome will be mapped out by the end of this year. [This prediction has come true.]

At the University of Utah, an artificial chromosome has been created that self-destructs on command if it is faulty or if it looks primitive to some future generation. I leave you to imagine what this could do and what the possibilities of such technologies are. . . .

The private sector is investing billions into biotechnology. Huge amounts of money are being made on the stock market. The manipulation of human beings seems to have no limits. This technology threatens the human species far more than abortion does. Abortion is a one-on-one destruction of a human being. What I am talking about today is a totality of changing the human species in defining what we are as humans. If a cow egg is deprived of its nucleus and a human nucleus has been put into that cow egg, now we have a hybrid of a cow and human that has been electrified and started to grow. What kind of person or organism is that going to be?

The geneticists, in short, are running wild. I am demanding Congress get involved in this to a much greater extent than it already has.

As the Human Genome Project crossed its finish line, there was surprisingly little public debate concerning the possible impact of the largest biology project ever undertaken: 1,110 biologists and computer scientists at sixteen laboratories in six countries over a period of thirteen years (and counting), at the cost of $250 million (and counting), mapping the precise chemical sequence that makes up the DNA in every cell of the human body. The project—reading and completing a working draft of 90 percent of the genome, the 3.2 billion chemical "letters" in human DNA, with 99.9 percent accuracy—was completed in mid-2000. Reports Sharon Begley in *Newsweek* magazine:

> With knowledge of our genetic code will come the power to re-engineer the human species. Biologists will be able to use the genome as a parts list—much as customers scour a list of china to replace broken plates—and may well let prospective parents choose their unborn child's traits. Scientists have solid leads on genes for specific temperaments, body builds, statures and cognitive abilities. And if anyone still believes that parents will recoil at playing God, and leave their babies' fate in the hands of nature, recall that couples have already created a frenzied market in eggs from Ivy League women.[8]

In his prize-winning book, *The Sun, the Genome, and the Internet: Tools of Scientific Revolution*, Dr. Freeman J. Dyson, Professor Emeritus of Physics at the Institute for Advanced Study, Princeton University, wisely observes:

> Many parents spend the greater part of their disposable income to send their children to private schools and universities, believing that education is the key to success. If, for a small fraction of the cost of higher education, parents could endow their children with superior genes, the demand for reprogenetics might become irresistible. Superior genes might give a

child the ability to become an Olympic figure-skating champion, or to be the chief executive officer of a company, or whatever else the ambitious parents might wish. Unfortunately, it would not be possible for the parents to obtain the informed consent of the child before undertaking the experiment. Nobody yet knows whether superior genes exist or how they might be identified. But the progress of knowledge of human genetics is rapid, and the technology of reprogenetics will not be far behind.[9]

"Today, we are more concerned about the abuse of reproductive freedom than about the vividness of *Brave New World*. Rather than being the cruel instrument of totalitarian government, eugenics has become transformed as people seek to fulfill their ambition to have the most treasured object—a healthy child," observes Dr. Roger Gosden, an early IVF pioneer and former colleague of Dr. Robert G. Edwards at Cambridge University. He adds:

> Over the centuries, we have secured food supplies, controlled epidemic diseases, and even managed from time to time to achieve political stability. In the twentieth century, couples became able to choose the number and timing of their children, and great advances were made in overcoming infertility. But reproduction is still a chancy business and often fails after an apparently good start or produces a less than perfect product. If the twentieth century was notable for fertility control, in the twenty-first century the emphasis of research will switch to producing a baby that is free from defects and attractive and arrives with perfect timing.[10]

Bill Joy, a widely renowned scientist and co-founder of computer technology firm Sun Microsystems, offers a considerably more sobering view of the far-reaching implications of twenty-first-century technologies:[11]

> What was different about the 20th century? Certainly, the technologies underlying the weapons of mass destruction (WMD)—nuclear, biological, and chemical (NBC)—were

powerful, and the weapons an enormous threat. But building nuclear weapons required, at least for a time, both access to rare—indeed, effectively unavailable—raw materials and highly protected information: biological and chemical weapons programs also tended to require large-scale activities.

The 21st-century technologies—genetics, nanotechnology, and robotics (GNR)—are so powerful that they can spawn whole new classes of accidents and abuses. Most dangerously, for the first time, these accidents and abuses are widely within the reach of individuals or small groups. They will not require large facilities or rare raw materials. Knowledge alone will enable the use of them.

Thus we have the possibility of not just weapons of mass destruction but of knowledge-enabled mass destruction (KMD), this destructiveness hugely amplified by the power of self-replication.

I think it is no exaggeration to say we are on the cusp of the further perfection of extreme evil, an evil whose possibility spreads well beyond that which weapons of mass destruction bequeathed to the nation-states, on to a terrible and surprising empowerment of extreme individuals.

Guarding, Protecting, Preserving Our Natural Design

I am not a physician or a philosopher who brings to this discussion advanced academic skills in the art of diagnosis or debate. Instead, I have written about these topics as a health educator and as a woman, in a voice strengthened by my conviction that the natural design of normal reproductive experience is worth guarding, protecting, and preserving. When I read the Psalms, I am particularly struck with the majesty and vulnerability of what it means to be created in God's image:

> O LORD, our Lord,
> how majestic is your name in all the earth!
> You have set your glory
> above the heavens.
> From the lips of children and infants
> you have ordained praise
> because of your enemies,

> *to silence the foe and the avenger.*
> *When I consider your heavens,*
> *the work of your fingers,*
> *the moon and the stars,*
> *which you have set in place,*
> *what is man that you are mindful of him,*
> *the son of man that you care for him?*
> *You made him a little lower than the heavenly beings*
> *and crowned him with glory and honor.*[12]

Technology often drowns out the sound of this symphony.

"A science-based culture, such as the present one, of necessity erodes and makes nonsense out of all sorts of bonds and connections which a Christian sees to be the case," says Princeton University theologian Paul Ramsey.[13] The reason for this, Ramsey explains, is directly related to our created identity:

> Men and women are created in covenant, to covenant, and for covenant. Creation is *toward* the love of Christ. Christians, therefore, will not readily admit that the energies of sex, for example, have any other primary *telos*, any other final end, than Jesus Christ. Rather, they will find in the strength of human sexual passion (beyond the obvious needs of procreation) an evident *telos* of acts of sexual love toward making real the meaning of man-womanhood, nurturing covenant-love between the parties, fostering their care for one another, prefiguring Christ's love for the Church. . . . *And in human procreativity out of the depths of human sexual love is prefigured God's own act of creation out of the profound mystery of his love revealed in Christ.* To put radically asunder what God joined together in parenthood when He made love procreative, to procreate beyond the sphere of love (artificial insemination by donor, for example, or making human life in a test tube), or to posit acts of sexual love beyond the sphere of responsible procreation (by definition, marriage), means a refusal of the image of God's creation in our own.[14]

The current level of reproductive technologies performed on women in this country attempts to redesign procreation through invasive ARTs. But instead of improving women's health, many of these medical treatments and techniques sabotage the physiological integrity of our bodies. Assisted reproductive technologies have opened the door to an ever-widening invasion of our natural design.

It is those who pay for medical care who usually can most influence change, not those who provide it. You and I can decide where and how to spend our health-care dollars—what hospitals to utilize, which physicians to visit, which preventative strategies to invest in, which medical treatments to give our consent to—and thus make a direct impact on health-care services and providers in our local communities. By educating ourselves about our bodies and becoming responsible about the health-care choices we make, we can avoid unnecessary invasive surgery and high-risk, low-yield medical treatments.[15]

For normal childbirth and well-woman gynecological care, for example, we can select midwives in order to receive care from highly skilled providers trained in the art of nurturing healthy laboring women. For breastfeeding assistance, we can contact lactation consultants to give us the advice and support we need for nursing our babies. For family planning, we can learn how to live in harmony with the natural rhythms and patterns of our bodies during each menstrual cycle. For fertility promotion, we can avoid unhealthful lifestyles, harmful contraceptive drugs and devices, sexually transmitted diseases, and delayed childbearing.

Infertility medicine presents its own set of unique challenges and dilemmas. *If a woman is having difficulty becoming pregnant, she should take time to assess her lifestyle and learn how to observe signs of fertility before resorting to medical therapy—if there are no unusual symptoms of reproductive disease or disability.*

Stress, diet, weight, age, exercise, and a woman's current health status all contribute to the ability to carry a baby. In addition, it is important to remember that many women have at least one or two anovulatory cycles per year (cycles in which menstruation occurs, but not ovulation) and that the average length of time it takes to conceive is eight months. Because infertility diagnosis and treatment often involves expensive procedures without guarantees of success, it is essential to proceed carefully when selecting a health-care provider or making decisions about infertility therapy.

A few years ago, I received a call from a woman who had spent over $7,000 on infertility treatment in the previous five months. She told me about being put on a fertility drug and the diagnostic tests she and her husband had endured. What angered me the most about this woman's story is that her physician had put her on this medication and performed a battery of diagnostic procedures but hadn't even asked basic questions about her stress level, diet, and exercise habits, or attitudes about marriage and family life. Neither had she been adequately taught to observe her body's signs of fertility—cervical mucus, cervical dilation, and basal body temperature—to determine when, and if, she was ovulating. In fact, the physician had not yet determined if ovulation was taking place.

As we talked, I discovered that this woman holds three jobs, travels out of town extensively, eats erratically, and describes herself as constantly under an incredible amount of stress. Nutritional therapy, ovulation awareness, and stress management had not occurred to her as possible resolutions to her difficulty in getting pregnant. Think about it: Doesn't it make sense to try this approach *before* bombarding one's body with hormones and surgery?

Another woman—a labor and delivery nurse—told me that at her first infertility appointment, her gynecologist had automatically prescribed Clomid when she told him she wasn't conceiving. Other than taking her history, he made no attempt to determine whether she was ovulating. She then told me of a friend whose ob/gyn immediately decided to perform a laparoscopy when she asked for help in conceiving. Clearly, the expense and risks of these procedures should provoke couples to consider in advance how much they are willing to spend or endure at the hands of an infertility specialist, as well as to find out the appropriate indications for specific procedures.

The Giver of Life

While writing this book, I took time out to visit the Rocky Mountains and climb to the top of a mountain. The path was lined by alpine tundra. After spending countless hours in medical libraries, I enjoyed being surrounded with the nonsynthetic reality of glacier-fed streams and ancient rock formations. The panoramic view surrounding me was thoroughly refreshing as I feasted on the beauty of snowy peaks rimming the horizon. I was reminded of the following verses:

> For you created my inmost being;
> you knit me together in my mother's womb.
> I praise you because I am fearfully and wonderfully made;
> your works are wonderful,
> I know that full well.[16]

It was awe-inspiring to realize that the God who created the sky and mountains made me too.

Several weeks later I ran into an article describing the nation's first IVF program in Norfolk, Virginia.[17] In it the author describes a sign with a subtle but significant message hanging on the clinic's waiting room wall. It reads: "They say babies are made in heaven, but we know better."

Yet the Bible says: "Know that the LORD Himself is God; it is He who has made us, and not we ourselves."[18] Children are gifts of God, not laboratory-designed creations. What reproductive technology delivers in cleverly designed packages is selective breeding, genetic diagnosis, embryo experimentation, and the medical control of life from the earliest moments—not babies. *No amount of technology can produce life.* That alone belongs to God to give.

Not surprisingly, one of the experimental projects conducted at the Norfolk clinic (now called the Jones Institute of Reproductive Medicine) was research on the abortion pill RU486.[19] My immediate reaction upon learning this fact was to ask myself why an *infertility* clinic would also be investigating contraception and abortion techniques. To say this is a conflict of interest is putting it mildly, unless one clearly understands that the "miraculous" results of infertility treatments are all the public is often allowed to see of these programs.

"We want to be able to develop to the fullest extent the research potential which lies in our program," said Dr. Howard Jones, Jr., the director of the clinic.[20] In the case of the Jones Clinic, this apparently means more than providing infertile couples with children.

In vitro fertilization, embryo transplants, and artificial wombs dehumanize conception. Commercialized programs further destroy the inherent design of procreation. The ends simply do not justify the means when it comes to attempts to make human beings. Says attorney Joseph J. Piccone:

> In vitro techniques are grossly careless toward human life. In addition to the risks to children born through such intervention, in vitro techniques also require the destruction of human embryos. . . .
>
> We should rejoice in the real progress of science, but must evaluate advances so that science truly serves humanity. The technical ability to do something does not itself justify the action. We've got to be able to reflect on our technology, or we will become victims of our short-term "success" and long-term failures.
>
> Poet e. e. cummings wrote that "a world of made is not a world of born." We have the ability to follow two different roads—one of respecting and enhancing human life, the other of reshaping and redefining it. This second choice is for the world of "made" in which life itself is mechanistic and impersonal. What is produced in the lab goes on to the courthouse, where it is just another issue in contract or property law.[21]

Which road will we choose?

Some are already making a difference, such as those who signed and submitted a summary statement to Congress titled "On Human Embryos and Stem Cell Research: An Appeal for Legally and Ethically Responsible Science and Public Policy."[22] The statement emphasized:

- Human embryonic stem cell research violates existing law and policy.
- Human embryonic stem cell research is unethical.
- Human embryonic stem cell research is scientifically unnecessary.

On August 23, 2000, the U.S. government issued new guidelines via the National Institutes of Health (NIH) permitting federal funding to finance research on human embryonic stem cells, despite the previous congressional ban on such funding. Kansas Senator Sam Brownback objected, "Destructive embryo research is illegal. Congress outlawed federal funding for harmful embryo research in 1996 and has maintained that prohibition. The ban is broad-based and specific; funds cannot be used for 'research in which a human embryo or embryos are destroyed, discarded or knowingly subjected to risk of injury or death.' The intent of Congress is clear."[23]

In an open letter to President Clinton and NIH Director Dr. Harold Varmus, Thomas Moore, Chairman and CEO of Cord Blood Registry, points out "that scientific research using embryonic cells is too great a leap to make when other viable and non-ethically controversial alternatives to scientific research into the wonders of stem cells exist." As Moore explains, umbilical cord blood, which is often discarded after the birth of a child, is a rich resource of readily available immature stem cells. Researchers have already found cord blood stem cells that have the ability to regenerate into heart capillary tissue. In fact, umbilical cord blood stem cells have shown superior qualities in comparison to bone marrow stem cells (which have the ability to regenerate into nerve, bone, liver, and other tissues) in the treatment of over thirty life-threatening diseases. The life materials used in embryonic studies are similar to those found in umbilical cord blood, but umbilical cord blood stem cells are a by-product of a new life— not the consequence of a destroyed one.

"The genesis of the call for embryonic research was based upon findings using bone marrow stem cells," Moore notes in the letter. "As cord blood possesses many superior qualities to bone marrow, and that the life ingredients of embryonic stem cells and cord blood are closely related, we urge you to look at the alternatives before pursuing the current course."[24]

Cord Blood Registry (CBR) is the world's largest cord blood stem cell bank. To date, over 20,000 babies throughout the United States have their cord blood stem cells entrusted to CBR.

I believe many people are willing to speak out who have not yet done so. Perhaps through prayer, informed community involvement, and/or appropriate legislative action, you too will choose to become actively involved. "We can and must find ways to help our fellow human beings triumph over life-destroying diseases. But we cannot do that by destroying lives ourselves," observes Senator Brownback. "We cannot secure a good life by ending the lives of others. There are other paths available—let us take them."[25]

May our voices ring out loudly and clearly to maintain that the wonder and majesty of God's good creation is worth protecting, guarding and preserving. We *can* make a difference in limiting the destructive techniques aimed at commercializing procreation and manipulating human life during its earliest stages.

Afterword

It might be going too far to say that the modern scientific movement was tainted from its birth, but I think it would be true to say that it was born in an unhealthy neighborhood and at an inauspicious hour. Its triumphs may have been too rapid and purchased at too high a price: reconsideration, and something like repentance, may be required.[1]

—C. S. LEWIS, *THE ABOLITION OF MAN*

When we discuss problems concerning adults and children, the National Institutes of Health is quite generally preferred. But when dealing with tiny fellows, especially the not-yet-born, the National Institute of Death finds some supporters. The reason for this divergence seems to lie in the question: Are they human or not? If already human, help and heal is the goal. If not yet human, discard and destroy is the solution.[2]

—DR. JEROME LEJEUNE

When one states that from the moment of conception one is dealing with a human being with certain inalienable rights, then one can be absolutely consistent in saying, "No abortion; no infanticide; no euthanasia."[3]

—DR. LEON KASS

W hen I wrote the first edition of *Without Moral Limits,* how could I have known that I was being uniquely prepared for a momentous family event? What I did not foresee during the long months of research and writing in 1988 and 1989 was that our oldest daughter Joanna would give birth to Abigail Elizabeth White, our first grandchild. A few years later came the incredible moment when I met Abigail for the first time as she slipped from my daughter's body into the cool air of a strangely hushed birthing room.

I will never forget that moment. How beautiful and precious our new granddaughter was! I was so proud of my daughter and son-in-law as they welcomed their firstborn ten hours after learning the life-changing news: A diagnostic ultrasound, ordered early in Joanna's labor to assess placental function, told us Abigail would be arriving with immediate medical needs, requiring her quick transfer to a nearby children's hospital and surgery. The last-minute diagnosis was hydrocephalus and spina bifida.

The research, prayer, and thinking that had gone into writing *Without Moral Limits* stood me in good stead during the first weeks of Abigail's life, and they remain with me still. Before Abigail was born, I knew in my mind what I believed about the value of each person's life. Now I know this truth by heart.

For nearly thirty years my husband, David, and I have been deeply committed to the public advocacy of persons with developmental disabilities and mental retardation. For David, this has meant investing the entirety of his professional life to full-time work in the MHMR field—from directing a large group home in Pontiac, Michigan, in the early seventies to his work as Georgia's director overseeing the state's mental health, mental retardation, and substance abuse programs in the nineties, to acting as the executive director of the Austin Travis County MHMR center here in Texas today. I cannot remember a time in our life together when we were not aware of our moral responsibility to speak and act on behalf of people who could not act and speak for themselves.

Welcoming Abigail into our family circle has made this awareness more personal, less theoretical. We are closer to both the pain and the joy experienced by someone whom many others have judged unworthy of life. The majority of babies who develop spina bifida very early in their lives, sometime around the fourth week of gestation, never make it to birth. If their mothers are provided the tests to detect the condition—typically an alpha-fetoprotein test followed by ultrasound imaging—they are aborted following prenatal diagnosis.

One of Abigail's doctors used to keep her picture as a reminder. Out of the thousands of children he had treated, hers was the only photograph on his desk. Abigail was his sole patient with spina bifida, the one person who "had made it."

She is a fragile survivor of an unseen holocaust, my granddaughter, and as yet is blissfully unaware of her special status in a world where being deemed "defective" too often is a death sentence. How can one possibly make sense of this terrible truth, given the advances modern medicine has made in treating children born with developmental and genetic disabilities such as spina bifida and Down syndrome?

Dr. Leon R. Kass observes:

> It is ironic that we should acquire the power to detect and eliminate the genetically unequal at a time when we have finally succeeded in removing much of the stigma and disgrace previously attached to victims of congenital illness, in providing them with improved care and support, and in preventing, by means of education, feelings of guilt on the part of their parents. One might even wonder whether the development of amniocentesis and prenatal diagnosis may represent a backlash against these same humanitarian and egalitarian tendencies in the practice of medicine, which, by helping to sustain to the age of reproduction persons with genetic disease has itself contributed to the increasing incidence of genetic disease, and with it, to increased pressures for genetic screening, genetic counseling, and genetic abortion.[4]

Dr. Kass adds:

> Any discussion of the ethical issues of genetic counseling and prenatal diagnosis is unavoidably haunted by a ghost called the morality of abortion. . . . The practice of abortion of the genetically defective will no doubt affect our view and our behavior toward those abnormals who escape the net of detection and abortion. A child with Down syndrome or with hemophilia or with muscular dystrophy born at a time when most of his fellow sufferers were destroyed prenatally is liable to be looked upon by the community as one unfit to be alive, as a second class (or even lower) human type.
>
> Precisely because the quality of the fetus is central to the decision to abort, the practice of genetic abortion has implications which go way beyond those raised by abortion in general. What may be at stake here is the belief in the radical moral equality of all human beings, the belief that all human beings

possess equally and independent of merit certain fundamental rights, one among which is, of course, the right to life.

To be sure, the belief that fundamental human rights belong equally to all human beings has been but an ideal, never realized, often ignored, sometimes shamelessly. Yet it has been perhaps the most powerful moral idea at work in the world for at least two centuries. It is this idea and ideal that animates most of the political and social criticism around the globe.[5]

Dr. Kass's words helped inform and shape my thinking long before "this idea and ideal" became more immediately real to us through our granddaughter's presence in our daily lives. Spending time with Abigail introduces us to new lessons in faith, and her very life tangibly affirms for us that nothing can happen to anyone without God's permission. Nothing. The ancient words of the prophet Isaiah have become even more meaningful to us as we have carefully considered this passage:

> Woe to him who quarrels with his Maker. . . .
> Does the clay say to the potter, "What are you making?"
> Does your work say, "He has no hands"?
> Woe to him who says to his father, "What have you begotten?"
>   or to his mother, "What have you brought to birth?"
> This is what the LORD says—
>   the Holy One of Israel, and its Maker:
> Concerning things to come,
>   do you question me about my children,
>   or give me orders about the work of my hands?
> It is I who made the earth and created mankind upon it.
> My own hands stretched out the heavens;
>   I marshaled their starry hosts.

ISAIAH 45:9-12

As I held my newborn granddaughter in my arms for the first time, I felt no fear or doubt concerning her Maker's sovereign design for her life. Though I had myriad concerns about the medical procedures she would require, the negative attitudes she would face, the physical challenges she would endure, I knew Abigail was unerringly protected by the one who had made her.

We didn't know in advance that Abigail would come into the world with multiple challenges to her central nervous system or that she would have a critical need for immediate surgery to close a small opening in her back caused by spina bifida. We didn't know what the future would hold for Abigail: How many more surgeries would she need? When would she be able to walk? To what degree would her condition affect her growth, her learning rate, her life expectancy? Abigail is now almost seven years old, and we still don't know the answers to those questions. None of us can see that far ahead.

Viewing Abigail's intrauterine image on the sonogram screen the day she was born revealed in stark terms the nature of her disability. As I stood in the back of the room behind the radiologist who was scanning Joanna's abdomen, I found the picture frightening because I had not met Abigail yet. I saw the problems, not the person. I am glad it was only a few hours before I looked into Abigail's blue eyes and spoke with her and only a few days before I held her in my arms and touched her soft skin, stroked her silky hair, and reveled in her new-born fragrance.

Perhaps it is especially true that when we come face to face with how little we know about the future—or the preborn person's abilities and disabilities—that we become more vulnerable to the power of a medical diagnosis, that we may be more likely to accept a doctor's proffered means of alleviating the pain and uncertainty involved. I understand this now. And that is why, more than ever, I believe the words in this book are worth heeding.

Abigail's presence in our lives reminds us where to look for help, wisdom, love, and strength—to rely less upon the things of this world and more on God. Taking life from her vantage point, we often find ourselves laughing more—and worrying less. Our hearts more freely open up to experiences we might otherwise miss. This is partly due to Abigail's genuine concern for others, that all might be well in the world. Since she is remarkably unattached to "things," she doesn't worry about accumulating possessions. Yet she never appears to be bored. This may be because, for Abigail, people are most important.

Arriving in the world with a damaged brain and spinal cord did
not limit our grandchild's ability to love us, nor did it prevent her from
getting to know her Creator. Though her sentences are typically short
or incomplete, somehow she has memorized and often says the entire
Lord's Prayer all by herself.

Being with Abigail reminds us to trust God with the burdens that
are His business, to look beyond our feelings of helplessness and frus-
tration for heavenly relief. Culturally valued forms of physical dex-
terity, intellectual ability, and social prowess are qualities that likely
will elude our granddaughter in the years to come. But while these
highly prized attributes may be missing, I see in Abigail God's strength
perfected in her weakness—the shining beauty of a tender heart
touched by His glory.

> *Where is the wise man? Where is the scholar? Where is the
> philosopher of this age? Has not God made foolish the wisdom of
> the world?. . . . But God chose the foolish things of the world to
> shame the wise; God chose the weak things of the world to shame
> the strong. He chose the lowly things of this world and the despised
> things—and the things that are not—to nullify the things that are,
> so that no one may boast before him.*
>
> 1 CORINTHIANS 1:20, 27-28

Appendix A

Vatican Statement on Noncoital Reproduction

The complete document issued by the Vatican on reproductive technology in February 1987 is presented here as a moral response to the gynetech philosophy. Since many Christians like myself were only informed of the Vatican's position through news headlines blaring "Vatican Condemns New Infertility Treatments," it seemed worthwhile to let people judge for themselves. What follows is a profoundly beautiful statement about the meaning of procreation and human life—a model for all Christians to consider thoughtfully and prayerfully.

This is the official Vatican English Language text of the "Instruction on Respect for Human Life in Its Origin and the Dignity of Procreation: Replies to Certain Questions of the Day" issued by the Congregation for the Doctrine of the Faith, dated February 22, 1987, and published March 10, 1987 (reprinted by permission of CRUX, Clarity Publishing, Inc., Albany, NY).

Vatican Statement

Instruction on Respect for Human Life and the Dignity of Procreation

FOREWORD

The Congregation for the Doctrine of the Faith has been approached by various episcopal conferences of individual bishops, by theologians, doctors, and scientists concerning biomedical techniques which make it possible to intervene in the initial phase of the life of a human being and in the very processes of procreation and their conformity with the principles of Catholic morality. The present Instruction, which is the result of wide consultation and in particular of a careful evaluation of the declarations made by episcopates, does not intend to repeat all the Church's teaching on the dignity of human life as it originates and on procreation, but to offer, in light of the previous teaching of the Magisterium, some specific replies to the main questions being asked in this regard.

The exposition is arranged as follows: An Introduction will recall the fundamental principles of an anthropological and moral character which are necessary for a proper evaluation of the problems and for working out replies to those questions; the first part will have as its subject respect for the human being from the first moment of his or her existence; the second part will deal with the moral questions raised by technical interventions on human procreation; the third part will offer some orientations on the relationships between moral law and civil law in terms of the respect due to human embryos and fetuses (see note) and as regards the legitimacy of techniques of artificial procreation.

Note: The terms "zygote," "pre-embryo," "embryo" and "fetus" can indicate in the vocabulary of biology successive stages of the development of a human being. The present Instruction makes free use of these terms, attributing to them an identical ethical relevance in order to designate the result (whether visible or not) of human generation from the first moment of its existence until birth. The reason for this usage is clarified by the text (cf. 11).

Introduction

1. BIOMEDICAL RESEARCH AND THE TEACHING OF THE CHURCH

The gift of life which God the Creator and Father has entrusted to man calls him to appreciate the inestimable value of what he has been given and to take responsibility for it: this fundamental principle must be placed at the center of one's reflection in order to clarify and solve the moral problems raised by artificial interventions on life as it originates and on the processes of procreation.

Thanks to the progress of the biological and medical sciences, man has at his disposal ever more effective therapeutic resources; but he can also acquire new powers with unforeseeable consequences over human life at its very beginning and in its first stages. Various procedures now make it possible to intervene not only in order to assist but also to dominate the processes of procreation. These techniques can enable man to "take in hand his own destiny," but they also expose him "to the temptation to go beyond the limits of a reasonable dominion over nature."[1] They might constitute progress in the service of man but they also involve serious risks. Many people are therefore expressing an urgent appeal that in interventions on procreation the values and rights of the human person be safeguarded. Requests for clarification and guidance are coming not only from the faithful, but also from those who recognize the Church as "an expert in humanity"[2] with a mission to serve the "civilization of love"[3] and of life.

The Church's Magisterium does not intervene on the basis of particular competence in the area of the experimental sciences; but having taken account of the data of research and technology, it intends to put forward, by virtue of its evangelical mission and apostolic duty, the moral teaching corresponding to the dignity of the person and to his or her integral vocation. It intends to do so by expounding the criteria of moral judgment as regards the applications of scientific research and technology, especially in relation to human life and its beginnings. These criteria are the respect, defense and promotion of man, his "primary and fundamental right" to life,[4] his dignity as a person who is endowed with a spiritual soul and with moral responsibility[5] and who is called to beatific communion with God.

The Church's intervention in this field is inspired also by the love which she owes to man, helping him to recognize and respect his rights and duties. This love draws from the fount of Christ's love: As she contemplates the mystery of the incarnate word, the Church also comes to understand the "mystery of man;"[6] by proclaiming the Gospel of salvation, she reveals to man his dignity and invites him to discover fully the truth of his own being. Thus the Church once more puts forward the divine law in order to accomplish the work of truth and liberation.

For it is out of goodness—in order to indicate the path of life—

that God gives human beings his commandments and the grace to observe them; and it is likewise out of goodness—in order to help them persevere along the same path—that God always offers to everyone his forgiveness. Christ has compassion in our weaknesses: He is our Creator and Redeemer. May his Spirit open men's hearts to the gift of God's peace and to an understanding of his precepts.

2. SCIENCE AND TECHNOLOGY AT THE SERVICE OF THE HUMAN PERSON

God created man in his own image and likeness: "Male and female he created them" (Gen. 1:27), entrusting to them the task of 'having dominion' over the earth" (Gen. 1:28). Basic scientific research and applied research constitute a significant expression of this dominion of man over creation. Science and technology are valuable resources for man when placed at his service and when they promote his integral development for the benefit of all; but they cannot of themselves show the meaning of existence and of human progress. Being ordered to man, who initiates and develops them, they draw from the person and his moral values the indication of their purpose and the awareness of their limits.

It would on the one hand be illusory to claim that scientific research and its applications are morally neutral; on the other hand one cannot derive criteria for guidance from mere technical efficiency, from research's possible usefulness to some at the expense of others or, worse still, from prevailing ideologies. Thus science and technology require for their own intrinsic meaning an unconditional respect for the fundamental criteria of the moral law: That is to say, they must be at the service of the human person, of his inalienable rights and his true and integral good according to the design and will of God.[7]

The rapid development of technological discoveries gives greater urgency to this need to respect the criteria just mentioned: Science without conscience can only lead to man's ruin. "Our era needs such wisdom more than bygone ages if the discoveries made by man are to be further humanized. For the future of the world stands in peril unless wiser people are forthcoming."[8]

3. ANTHROPOLOGY AND PROCEDURES IN THE BIOMEDICAL FIELD

Which moral criteria must be applied in order to clarify the problems posed today in the field of biomedicine? The answer to this question presupposes a proper idea of the nature of the human person in his bodily dimension. For it is only in keeping with his true nature that the human person can achieve self-realization as a "unified totality;"[9] and this nature is at the same time corporal and spiritual. By virtue of its substantial union with a spiritual soul, the human body cannot be considered as a mere complex of tissues, organs and functions, nor can it be evaluated in the same way as the body of animals; rather it is a constitutive part of the person, who manifests and expresses himself through it.

The natural moral law expresses and lays down the purposes, rights and duties which are based upon the bodily and spiritual nature of the human person. Therefore this law cannot be thought of as simply a set of norms on the biological level; rather it must be defined as the rational order whereby man is called by the Creator to direct and regulate his life and actions and in particular to make use of his own body.[10]

A first consequence can be deduced from these principles: an intervention on the human body affects not only the tissues, the organs and their functions, but also involves the person himself on different levels. It involves, therefore, perhaps in an implicit but nonetheless real way, a moral significance and responsibility. Pope John Paul II forcefully reaffirmed this to the World Medical Association when he said: "Each human person, in his absolute singularity, is constituted not only by his spirit, but by his body as well. Thus, in the body and through the body, one touches the person himself in his concrete reality. To respect the dignity of man consequently amounts to safeguarding this identity of the man '*corpore et anima unus,*' as the Second Vatican Council says (*Gaudium et Spes,* 14.1). It is on the basis of this anthropological vision that one is to find the fundamental criteria for decision making in the case of procedures which are not strictly therapeutic, as, for example, those aimed at the improvement of the human biological condition."[11]

Applied biology and medicine work together for the integral good

of human life when they come to the aid of a person stricken by illness and infirmity and when they respect his or her dignity as a creature of God. No biologist or doctor can reasonably claim, by virtue of
his scientific competence, to be able to decide on people's origin and
destiny. This norm must be applied in a particular way in the field of
sexuality and procreation, in which man and woman actualize the fundamental values of love and life.

God, who is love and life, has inscribed in man and woman the
vocation to share in a special way in his mystery of personal communion and in his work as Creator and Father.[12] For this reason marriage
possesses specific goods and values in its union and in procreation
which cannot be likened to those existing in lower forms of life. Such
values and meanings are the personal order and determine from the
moral point of view the meaning and limits of artificial interventions
on procreation and on the origin of human life. These interventions
are not to be rejected on the grounds that they are artificial. As such,
they bear witness to the possibilities of the art of medicine. But they
must be given a moral evaluation in reference to the dignity of the
human person, who is called to realize his vocation from God to the
gift of love and the gift of life.

4. FUNDAMENTAL CRITERIA FOR A MORAL JUDGMENT

The fundamental values connected with the techniques of artificial
human procreation are two: the life of the human being called into
existence and the special nature of the transmission of human life in
marriage. The moral judgment on such methods of artificial procreation must therefore be formulated in reference to these values.

Physical life, with which the course of human life in the world
begins, certainly does not itself contain the whole of a person's value
nor does it represent the supreme good of man, who is called to eter-
nal life. However it does constitute in a certain way the "fundamental
value of life" precisely because upon this physical life all the other values of the person are based and developed.[13] The inviolability of the
innocent human being's right to life "from the moment of conception

until death"[14] is a sign and requirement of the inviolability of the person to whom the Creator has given the gift of life.

By comparison with the transmission of other forms of life in the universe, the transmission of human life has a special character of its own, which derives from the special nature of the human person. "The transmission of human life is entrusted by nature to a personal and conscious act and as such is subject to the all-holy laws of God: immutable and inviolable laws which must be recognized and observed. For this reason one cannot use means and follow methods which could be licit in the transmission of the life of plants and animals."[15]

Advances in technology have now made it possible to procreate apart from sexual relations through the meeting "in vitro" of the germ cells previously taken from the man and woman. But what is technically possible is not for that very reason morally admissible. Rational reflection on the fundamental values of life and of human procreation is therefore indispensable for formulating a moral evaluation of such technological interventions on a human being from the first stages of his development.

5. TEACHINGS OF THE MAGISTERIUM

On its part, the Magisterium of the Church offers to human reason in this field too the light of revelation: The doctrine concerning man taught by the Magisterium contains many elements which throw light on the problems being faced here.

From the moment of conception, the life of every human being is to be respected in an absolute way because man is the only creature on earth that God has "wished from himself,"[16] and the spiritual soul of each man is "immediately created" by God;[17] his whole being bears the image of the Creator. Human life is sacred because from its beginning it involves "the creative action of God,"[18] and it remains forever in a special relationship with the Creator, who is its sole end.[19] God alone is the Lord of life from its beginning until its end: no one can, in any circumstance, claim for himself the right to destroy directly an innocent human being.[20]

Human procreation requires on the part of the spouses responsible collaboration with the fruitful love of God;[21] the gift of human life must be actualized in marriage through the specific and exclusive acts of husband and wife, in accordance with the laws inscribed in their persons and in their union.[22]

I. RESPECT FOR HUMAN EMBRYOS

Careful reflection on this teaching of the Magisterium and on the evidence of reason, as mentioned above, enables us to respond to the numerous moral problems posed by technical interventions upon the human being in the first phases of his life and upon the processes of his conception.

1. *What respect is due the human embryo, taking into account his nature and identity?* The human being must be respected—as a person—from the very first instant of his existence. The implications of procedures of artificial fertilization has made possible various interventions upon embryos and human fetuses. The aims pursued are of various kinds: Diagnostic and therapeutic, scientific and commercial. From all of this, serious problems arise. Can one speak of a right to experimentation upon human embryos for the purpose of scientific research? What norms or laws should be worked out with regard to this matter? The response to these problems presupposes a detailed reflection on the nature and specific identity—the word "status" is used—of the human embryo itself.

At the Second Vatican Council, the Church for her part presented once again to modern man her constant and certain doctrine according to which: "Life once conceived, must be protected with the utmost care; abortion and infanticide are abominable crimes."[23] More recently, the Charter of the Rights of the Family, published by the Holy See, confirmed that "human life must be absolutely respected and protected from the moment of conception."[24]

This congregation is aware of the current debates concerning the beginning of human life, concerning the individuality of the human being, and concerning the identity of the human person. The congregation recalls the teachings found in the Declaration on Procured Abortion:

"From the time that the ovum is fertilized, a new life is begun which is neither that of the father nor of the mother; it is rather the life of a new human being with his own growth. It would never be made human if it were not human already. To this perpetual evidence . . . modern genetic science brings valuable confirmation. It has demonstrated that, from the first instant, the program is fixed as to what this living being will be: a man, this individual man with his characteristic aspects already well determined. Right from fertilization is begun the adventure of a human life, and each of its great capacities requires time . . . to find its place and to be in a position to act."[25]

This teaching remains valid and is further confirmed, if confirmation were needed, by recent findings of human biological science which recognize that in the zygote (the cell produced when the nuclei of the two gametes have fused) resulting from fertilization, the biological identity of a new human individual is already constituted.

Certainly no experimental datum can be in itself sufficient to bring us to the recognition of a spiritual soul; nevertheless, the conclusions of science regarding the human embryo provide a valuable indication for discerning by the use of reason a personal presence at the moment of this first appearance of a human life: How could a human individual not be a human person? The Magisterium has not expressly committed itself to an affirmation of a philosophical nature, but it constantly reaffirms the moral condemnation of any kind of procured abortion. This teaching has not been changed and is unchangeable.[26]

Thus the fruit of human generation from the first moment of its existence, that is to say, from the moment the zygote has formed, demands the unconditional respect that is morally due to the human being in his bodily and spiritual totality. The human being is to be respected and treated as a person from the moment of conception, and therefore from that same moment his rights as a person must be recognized, among which in the first place is the inviolable right of every innocent human being to life.

This doctrinal reminder provides the fundamental criterion for the solution of the various problems posed by the development of the biomedical sciences in this field: Since the embryo must be treated as a person, it must also be defended in its integrity, tended and cared for, to the extent possible, in the same way as any other human being as far as medical assistance is concerned.

2. *Is prenatal diagnosis morally licit?* If prenatal diagnosis respects the life and integrity of the embryo and the human fetus and is directed toward its safeguarding or healing as an individual, then the answer is affirmative.

For prenatal diagnosis makes it possible to know the condition of the embryo and of the fetus when still in the mother's womb. It permits or makes it possible to anticipate earlier and more effectively, certain therapeutic, medical or surgical procedures.

Such diagnosis is permissible, with the consent of the parents after they have been adequately informed, if the methods employed safeguard the life and integrity of the embryo and the mother, without subjecting them to disproportionate risks.[27] But this diagnosis is gravely opposed to the moral law when it is done with the thought of possibly inducing an abortion depending upon the results: A diagnosis which shows the existence of a malformation or hereditary illness must not be the equivalent of a death sentence. Thus a woman would be committing a gravely illicit act if she were to request such a diagnosis with the deliberate intention of having an abortion should the results confirm the existence of a malformation or abnormality. The spouse or relatives of anyone else would similarly be acting in a manner contrary to the moral law if they were to counsel or impose such a diagnostic procedure on the expectant mother with the same intention of possibly proceeding to an abortion. So too the specialist would be guilty of illicit collaboration if, in conducting the diagnosis and in communicating its results, he were deliberately to contribute to establishing or favoring a link between prenatal diagnosis and abortion.

In conclusion, any directive or program of the civil and health authorities or of scientific organizations which in any way were to favor a link between prenatal diagnosis and abortion, or which were to go as far as directly to induce expectant mothers to submit to prenatal diagnosis planned for the purpose of eliminating fetuses which are affected by malformations or which are carriers of hereditary illness, is to be condemned as a violation of the unborn child's right to life and as an abuse of the prior rights and duties of the spouses.

3. *Are therapeutic procedures carried out on the human embryo licit?* As with all medical interventions on patients, one must uphold as licit procedures carried out on the human embryo which respect the life and integrity of the embryo and do not involve disproportionate risks for it, but are directed toward its healing, the improvement of its condition of health or its individual survival.

Whatever the type of medical, surgical or other therapy, the free and informed consent of the parents is required, according to the deontological rules followed in the case of children. The application of this moral principle may call for delicate and particular precautions in case of embryonic or fetal life.

The legitimacy and criteria of such procedures have been clearly stated by Pope John Paul II: "A strictly therapeutic intervention whose explicit objective is the healing of various maladies such as those stemming from chromosomal defects will, in principle, be considered desirable, provided it is directed to the true promotion of the personal well-being of the individual without doing harm to his integrity or worsen his conditions of life. Such an intervention would indeed fall within the logic of the Christian moral tradition."[28]

4. *How is one to evaluate morally research and experimentation (see note) on human embryos and fetuses?* Medical research must refrain from operations on live embryos, unless there is a moral certainty of not causing harm to the life or integrity of the unborn child and the mother, and on condition that the parents have given their free and informed consent to the procedure. It follows that all research, even when limited to the simple observation of the embryo, would become illicit were it to involve risk to the embryo's physical integrity or life by reason of the methods used or the effects induced.

As regards experimentation, and presupposing the general distinction between experimentation for purposes which are not directly therapeutic and experimentation which is clearly therapeutic for the subject himself, in the case in point one must also distinguish between experimentation carried out on embryos which are still alive and experimentation carried out on embryos which are dead. If the embryos are living, whether viable or not, they must be respected just like any other human person; experimentation on embryos which is not directly therapeutic is illicit.[29]

No objective, even though noble in itself such as a foreseeable advantage to science, to other human beings or to society, can in any way justify experimentation on living human embryos or fetuses, whether viable or not, either inside or outside the mother's womb. The informed consent ordinarily required for clinical experimentation on adults cannot be granted by the parents, who may not freely dispose of the physical integrity or life of the unborn child. Moreover, experimentation on embryos and fetuses always involves risk, and indeed in most cases it involves the certain expectation of harm to their physical integrity or even their death.

To use human embryos or fetuses as the object or instrument of experimentation constitutes a crime against their dignity as human beings having a right to the same respect that is due to the child already born and to every human person.

The Charter of the Rights of the Family published by the Holy See affirms: "Respect for the dignity of the human being excludes all experimental manipulation or exploitation of the human embryo."[30] The practice of keeping alive human embryos "in vivo" or "in vitro" for experimental or commercial purposes is totally opposed to human dignity.

In the case of experimentation that is clearly therapeutic, namely, when it is a matter of experimental forms of therapy used for the benefit of the embryo itself in a final attempt to save its life and in the absence of other reliable forms of therapy, recourse to drugs or procedures not yet fully tested can be licit.[31]

The corpses of human embryos and fetuses, whether they have been deliberately aborted or not, must be respected just as the remains of other human beings. In particular, they cannot be subjected to mutilation or to autopsies if their death has not yet been verified and without the consent of the parents or of the mother. Furthermore, the moral requirements must be safeguarded that there be no complicity in deliberate abortion and that the risk of scandal be avoided. Also, in the case of dead fetuses, as for the corpses of adult persons, all commercial trafficking must be considered illicit and should be prohibited.

Note: Since the terms "research" and "experimentation" are often used equivalently and ambiguously, it is deemed necessary to specify the exact meaning given them in this document.

a) By "research" is meant any inductive-deductive process which aims at promoting the systematic observation of a given phenomenon in the human field or at verifying a hypothesis arising from previous observations.

b) By "experimentation" is meant any research in which the human being (in the various stages of his existence: embryo, fetus, child or adult) represents the object through which or upon which one intends to verify the effect, at present unknown or not sufficiently known, of a given treatment (e.g., pharmacological, teratogenic, surgical, etc.).

5. *How is one to evaluate morally the use for research purposes of embryos obtained by fertilization "in vitro?"* Human embryos obtained "in vitro" are human beings and subjects with rights: Their dignity and right to life must be respected from the first moment of their existence. It is immoral to produce human embryos destined to be exploited as disposable "biological material."

In the usual practice of "in vitro" fertilization, not all of the embryos are transferred to the woman's body; some are destroyed. Just as the Church condemns induced abortion, so also she forbids acts against the life of these human beings. It is a duty to condemn the particular gravity of the voluntary destruction of human embryos obtained "in vitro" for the sole purpose of research, either by means of artificial insemination or by means of "twin fission." By acting in this way, the researcher usurps the place of God; and, even though he may be unaware of this, he sets himself up as the master of the destiny of others inasmuch as he arbitrarily chooses whom he will allow to live and whom he will send to death and kills defenseless human beings.

Methods of observation or experimentation which damage or impose grave and disproportionate risks upon embryos obtained "in vitro" are morally illicit for the same reasons. Every human being is to be respected for himself and cannot be reduced in worth to a pure and simple instrument for the advantage of others. It is therefore not in conformity with the moral law deliberately to expose to death human embryos obtained "in vitro." In consequence of the fact that they have been produced "in vitro," those embryos which are not transferred into the body of the mother and are called "spare" are exposed to an absurd fate, with no possibility of their being offered safe means of survival which can be licitly pursued.

6. *What judgment should be made on other procedures of manipulating embryos connected with the "techniques of human reproduction?"* Techniques of fertilization "in vitro" can open the way to other forms of biological and genetic manipulation of human embryos, such as attempts or plans for fertilization between human and animal gametes and the gestation of human embryos in the uterus of animals, or the hypothesis or project of constructing artificial uteruses for the human embryo. These procedures are contrary to the human dignity proper to the embryo, and at the same time they are contrary to the right of every person to be conceived and to be born within marriage and from marriage.[32] Also, attempts or hypotheses for obtaining a human being without any connection with sexuality through "twin fission," cloning or parthenogenesis are to be considered contrary to the moral law, since they are in opposition to the dignity both of human procreation and of the conjugal union.

The freezing of embryos, even when carried out in order to preserve the life of the embryo—cyopreservation—constitutes an offense against the respect due to human beings by exposing them to grave risks of death or harm to their physical integrity and depriving them, at least temporarily, of maternal shelter and gestation, thus placing them in a situation in which further offenses and manipulation are possible.

Certain attempts to influence chromosomic or genetic inheritance are not therapeutic, but are aimed at producing human beings selected according to sex or other predetermined qualities. These manipulations are contrary to the personal dignity of the human being and his or her integrity and identity. Therefore in no way can they be justified on the grounds of possible beneficial consequences for future humanity.[33] Every person must be respected for himself. In this consists the dignity and right of every human being from his or her beginning.

II. INTERVENTIONS UPON HUMAN PROCREATION

By "artificial procreation" or "artificial fertilization" are understood here the different technical procedures directed toward obtaining a human conception in a manner other than the sexual union of man and woman. This Instruction deals with fertilization of an ovum in a test tube ("in vitro" fertilization) and artificial insemination through transfer into the woman's genital tracts of previously collected sperm.

A preliminary point for the moral evaluation of such technical procedures is constituted by the consideration of the circumstances and consequences which those procedures involve in relation to the respect due the human embryo. Development of the practice of "in vitro" fertilization has required innumerable fertilizations and destructions of human embryos. Even today the usual practice presupposes a hyperovulation on the part of the woman: A number of ova are withdrawn, fertilized and then cultivated "in vitro" for some days. Usually not all are transferred into the genital tracts of the woman; some embryos, generally called "spare," are destroyed or frozen. On occasion, some of the implanted embryos are sacrificed for various eugenic, economic or psychological reasons. Such deliberate destruction of human beings or their utilization for different purposes to the detriment of their integrity and life is contrary to the doctrine on procured abortion already recalled.

The connection between "in vitro" fertilization and the voluntary destruction of human embryos occurs too often. This is significant: Through these procedures, with apparently contrary purposes, life and death are subjected to the decision of man, who thus sets himself up as the giver of life and death by decree. This dynamic of violence and domination may remain unnoticed by those very individuals who, in wishing to utilize this procedure, become subject to it themselves. The facts recorded and the cold logic which links them must be taken into consideration for a moral judgment on "in vitro" fertilization and embryo transfer: The abortion mentality which has made this procedure possible thus leads, whether one wants it or not, to man's domination over the life and death of his fellow human beings and can lead to a system of radical eugenics.

Nevertheless, such abuses do not exempt one from a further and thorough ethical study of the techniques of artificial procreation considered in themselves, abstracting as far as possible from the destruction of embryos produced "in vitro."

The present Instruction will therefore take into consideration in the first place the problems posed by heterologous artificial fertilization (II, 1-3)(see Note 1), and subsequently those linked with homologous artificial fertilization (II, 4-6)(see Note 2).

Note 1: By the term "heterologous artificial fertilization" or "procreation," the Instruction means techniques used to obtain a human conception artificially by the use of gametes coming from at least one donor other than the spouses who are joined in marriage. Such techniques can be of two types:

a) Heterologous "in vitro" fertilization and embryo transfer: the technique used to obtain a human conception through the meeting "in vitro" of gametes taken from at least one donor other than the two spouses joined in marriage.

b) Heterologous artificial insemination: the technique used to obtain a human conception through the transfer into the genital tracts of the woman of the sperm previously collected from a donor other than the husband.

Note 2: By "artificial homologous fertilization" or "procreation," the Instruction means the technique used to obtain a human conception using the gametes of the two spouses joined in marriage. Homologous artificial fertilization can be carried out by two different methods:

a) Homologous "in vitro" fertilization and embryo transfer: the technique used to obtain a human conception through the meeting "in vitro" of the gametes of the spouses joined in marriage.

b) Homologous artificial insemination: the technique used to obtain a human conception through the transfer into the genital tracts of a married woman of the sperm previously collected from her husband.

Before formulating an ethical judgment on each of these procedures, the principles and values which determine the moral evaluation of each of them will be considered.

A. Heterologous Artificial Fertilization

1. *Why must human procreation take place in marriage?* Every human being is always to be accepted as a gift and blessing of God. However, from the moral point of view a truly responsible procreation vis-à-vis the unborn child must be the fruit of marriage.

For human procreation has specific characteristics by virtue of the personal dignity of the parents and of the children: The procreation of a new person, whereby the man and the woman collaborate with the power of the Creator, must be the fruit and the sign of the mutual self-giving of the spouses, of their love and of their fidelity.[34] The fidelity of the spouses in the unity of marriage involves reciprocal respect of their right to become a father and a mother only through each other.

The child has the right to be conceived, carried in the womb, brought into the world and brought up within marriage: It is through the secure and recognized relationship to his own parents that the child can discover his own identity and achieve his own proper human development.

The parents find in their child a confirmation and completion of their reciprocal self-giving: The child is the living image of their love, concrete expression of the paternity and maternity.[35]

By reason of the vocation and social responsibilities of the person, the good of the children and of the parents contributes to the good of civil society; the vitality and stability of society require that children come into the world within a family and that the family be firmly based on marriage.

The tradition of the church and anthropological reflection recognize in marriage and in its indissoluble unity the only setting worthy of truly responsible procreation.

2. *Does heterologous artificial fertilization conform to the dignity of the couple and to the truth of marriage?* Through "in vitro" fertilization and embryo transfer and heterologous artificial insemination human

conception is achieved through the fusion of gametes of at least one donor other than the spouses who are united in marriage. Heterologous artificial fertilization is contrary to the unity of marriage, to the dignity of the spouses, to the vocation proper to parents, and to the child's right to be conceived and brought into the world in marriage and from marriage.[36]

Respect for the unity of marriage and for conjugal fidelity demands that the child be conceived in marriage; the bond existing between husband and wife accords the spouses, in an objective and inalienable manner, the exclusive right to become father and mother solely through each other.[37]

Recourse to the gametes of a third person in order to have sperm or ovum available constitutes a violation of the reciprocal commitment of the spouses and a grave lack in regard to that essential property of marriage which is its unity.

Heterologous artificial fertilization violates the right of the child: It deprives him of his filial relationship with his parental origins and can hinder the maturing of his personal identity. Furthermore it offends the common vocation of the spouses who are called to fatherhood and motherhood. It objectively deprives conjugal fruitfulness of its unity and integrity; it brings about and manifests a rupture between genetic parenthood, gestational parenthood and responsibility for upbringing. Such damage to the personal relationships within the family has repercussions on civil society: What threatens the unity and stability of the family is a source of dissension, disorder and injustice in the whole of social life.

These reasons lead to a negative moral judgment concerning heterologous artificial fertilization: Consequently, fertilization of a married woman with the sperm of a donor different from her husband and fertilization with the husband's sperm of an ovum not coming from his wife are morally illicit. Furthermore, the artificial fertilization of a woman who is unmarried or a widow, whoever the donor may be, cannot be morally justified.

The desire to have a child and the love between spouses who long to obviate a sterility which cannot be overcome in any other way constitute understandable motivations, but subjectively good intentions do not render heterologous artificial fertilization conformable to the objective and inalienable properties of marriage or respectful of the rights of the child and of the spouses.

3. *Is "surrogate" (see note) motherhood morally licit?* No, for the same reasons which lead one to reject heterologous artificial fertilization: For it is contrary to the unity of marriage and to the dignity of the procreation of the human person.

Surrogate motherhood represents an objective failure to meet the obligations of maternal love, of conjugal fidelity and of responsible motherhood; it offends the dignity and the right of the child to be conceived, carried in the womb, brought into the world and brought up by his own parents: it sets up, to the detriment of families, a division between the physical, psychological and moral elements which constitute those families.

Note: By "surrogate mother" the Instruction means:

a) The woman who carries in pregnancy an embryo implanted in her uterus and who is genetically a stranger to the embryo because it has been obtained through the union of the gametes of "donors." She carries the pregnancy with a pledge to surrender the baby once it is born to the party who commissioned or made the agreement for the pregnancy.

b) The woman who carries in pregnancy an embryo to whose procreation she has contributed the donation of her own ovum, fertilized through the insemination with the sperm of a man other than her husband. She carries the pregnancy with a pledge to surrender the child once it is born to the party who commissioned or made the agreement for the pregnancy.

B. Homologous Artificial Fertilization

Since heterologous artificial fertilization has been declared unacceptable, the question arises of how to evaluate morally the process of homologous artificial fertilization: "in vitro" fertilization and embryo transfer and artificial insemination between husband and wife. First a question of principle must be clarified.

4. *What connection is required from the moral point of view between procreation and the conjugal act?*

a) The Church's teaching on marriage and human procreation affirms the "inseparable connection, willed by God and unable to be broken by man on his own initiative, between the two meanings of the conjugal act: the unitive meaning and the procreative meaning. Indeed, by its intimate structure the conjugal act, while most closely uniting husband and wife, capacitates them for the generation of new lives according to the laws inscribed in the very being of man and of woman."[38] This principle, which is based upon the nature of marriage and the intimate connection of the goods of marriage, has well-known consequences on the level of responsible fatherhood and motherhood. "By safeguarding both these essential aspects, the unitive and the procreative, the conjugal act preserves in its fullness the sense of true mutual love and its ordination toward man's exalted vocation to parenthood."[39]

The same doctrine concerning the link between the meanings of the conjugal act and between the goods of marriage throws light on the moral problem of homologous artificial fertilization, since "it is never permitted to separate those different aspects to such a degree as positively to exclude either the procreative intention or the conjugal relation."[40]

Contraception deliberately deprives the conjugal act of its openness to procreation and in this way brings about a voluntary dissociation of the ends of marriage. Homologous artificial fertilization, in seeking a procreation which is not the fruit of a specific act of conjugal union, objectively effects an analogous separation between the goods and the meaning of marriage.

Thus, fertilization is licitly sought when it is the result of a "conjugal act which is per se suitable for the generation of children, to which marriage is ordered by its nature and by which the spouses become one flesh."[41] But from the moral point of view procreation is deprived of its proper perfection when it is not desired as the fruit of the conjugal act, that is to say, of the specific act of the spouses' union.

b) The moral value of the intimate link between the goods of marriage and between the meanings of the conjugal act is based upon the unity of the human being, a unity involving body and spiritual soul.[42] Spouses mutually express their personal love in the "language of the body," which clearly involves both "spousal meanings" and parental ones.[43] The conjugal act by which the couple mutually express their self-gift at the same time expresses openness to the gift of life. It is an act that is inseparably corporal and spiritual. It is in their bodies and through their bodies that the spouses consummate their marriage and are able to become father and mother. In order to respect the language of their bodies and their natural generosity, the conjugal union must take place with respect for its openness to procreation; and the procreation of a person must be the fruit and the result of married love. The origin of the human being thus follows from a procreation that is "linked to the union, not only biological but also spiritual, of the parents, made one by the bond of marriage."[44] Fertilization achieved outside the bodies of the couple remains by this very fact deprived of the meanings and the values which are expressed in the language of the body and in the union of human persons.

c) Only respect for the link between the meanings of the conjugal act and respect for the unity of the human being make possible procreation in conformity with the dignity of the person. In his unique and unrepeatable origin, the child must be respected and recognized as equal in personal dignity to those who give him life. The human person must be accepted in his parents' act of union and love; the generation of a child must therefore be the fruit of the mutual giving[45] which is realized in the conjugal act wherein the spouses cooperate as servants and not as masters in the work of the Creator, who is love.[46]

In reality, the origin of a human person is the result of an act of giving. The one conceived must be the fruit of his parents' love. He cannot be desired or conceived as the product of an intervention of medical or biological techniques; that would be equivalent to reducing him to an object of scientific technology. No one may subject the coming of a child into the world to conditions of technical efficiency which are to be evaluated according to standards of control and dominion.

The moral relevance of the link between the meanings of the conjugal act and between the goods of marriage, as well as the unity of the human being and the dignity of his origin, demand that the pro-creation of a human person be brought about as the fruit of the con-jugal act specific to the love between spouses, the link between procreation and the conjugal act is thus shown to be of great impor-tance on the anthropological and moral planes, and it throws light on the positions of the Magisterium with regard to homologous artificial fertilization.

5. *Is homologous "in vitro" fertilization morally licit?* The answer to this question is strictly dependent on the principles just mentioned. Certainly one cannot ignore the legitimate aspirations of sterile cou-ples. For some, recourse to homologous "in vitro" fertilization and embryo transfer appears to be the only way of fulfilling their sincere desire for a child. The question is asked whether the totality of con-jugal life in such situations is not sufficient to ensure the dignity proper to human procreation. It is acknowledged that "in vitro" fer-tilization and embryo transfer certainly cannot supply for the absence of sexual relations[47] and cannot be preferred to the specific acts of con-jugal union, given the risks involved for the child and the difficulties of the procedure. But it is asked whether, when there is no other way of overcoming the sterility which is a source of suffering, homologous "in vitro" fertilization may not constitute an aid, if not a form of ther-apy, whereby its moral licitness could be admitted.

The desire for a child—or at least an openness to the transmission of life—is a necessary prerequisite from the moral point of view for responsible human procreation. But this good intention is not suffi-cient for making a positive moral evaluation of "in vitro" fertilization between spouses. The process of "in vitro" fertilization and embryo transfer must be judged in itself and cannot borrow its definitive moral quality from the totality of conjugal life of which it becomes part nor from the conjugal acts which may precede or follow it.[48]

It has already been recalled that in the circumstances in which it is regularly practiced, "in vitro" fertilization and embryo transfer involves the destruction of human beings, which is something con-trary to the doctrine on the illicitness of abortion previously men-tioned.[49] But even in a situation in which every precaution were taken to avoid the death of human embryos, homologous "in vitro" fertilization and embryo transfer dissociates from the conjugal act the actions which are directed to human fertilization. For this reason the very nature of homologous "in vitro" fertilization and embryo transfer also must be taken into account, even abstracting from the link with procured abortion.

Homologous "in vitro" fertilization and embryo transfer is brought about outside the bodies of the couple through actions of third parties whose competence and technical activity determine the success of the procedure. Such fertilization entrusts the life and identity of the embryo into the power of doctors and biologists and establishes the domination of technology over the origin and destiny of the human person. Such a relationship of domination is in itself contrary to the dignity and equality that must be common to parents and children.

Conception "in vitro" is the result of the technical action which presides over fertilization. Such fertilization is neither in fact achieved nor positively willed as the expression and fruit of a specific act of the conjugal union. In homologous "in vitro" fertilization and embryo transfer, therefore, even if it is considered in the context of de facto existing sexual relations, the generation of the human person is objectively deprived of its proper perfection: namely, that of being the result and fruit of a conjugal act in which the spouses can become "cooperators with God for giving life to a new person."[50]

These reasons enable us to understand why the act of conjugal love is considered in the teaching of the Church as the only setting worthy of human procreation. For the same reasons the so-called simple case, i.e., a homologous "in vitro" fertilization and embryo transfer procedure that is free of any compromise with the abortive practice of destroying embryos and with masturbation, remains a technique which is morally illicit because it deprives human procreation of the dignity which is proper and connatural to it.

Certainly, homologous "in vitro" fertilization and embryo transfer fertilization is not marked by all that ethical negativity found in extraconjugal procreation; the family and marriage continue to constitute the setting for the birth and upbringing of the children. Nevertheless, in conformity with the traditional doctrine relating to the goods of marriage and the dignity of the person, the Church remains opposed from the moral point of view to homologous "in vitro" fertilization. Such fertilization is in itself illicit and in opposition to the dignity of procreation and of the conjugal union, even when everything is done to avoid the death of the human embryo.

Although the manner in which human conception is achieved with "in vitro" fertilization and embryo transfer cannot be approved, every child which comes into the world must in any case be accepted as a living gift of the divine Goodness and must be brought up with love.

6. *How is homologous artificial insemination to be evaluated from the moral point of view?* Homologous artificial insemination within marriage cannot be admitted except for those cases in which the technical means is not a substitute for the conjugal act but serves to facilitate and to help so that the act attains its natural purpose.

The teaching of the Magisterium on this point has already been stated.[51] This teaching is not an expression of particular historical circumstances, but is based on the Church's doctrine concerning the connection between the conjugal union and procreation and on a consideration of the personal nature of the conjugal act and of human procreation. "In its natural structure, the conjugal act is a personal action, a simultaneous and immediate cooperation on the part of the husband and wife, which by the very nature of the agents and the proper nature of the act is the expression of the mutual gift which according to the words of Scripture, brings about union 'in one flesh.'"[52] Thus moral conscience "does not necessarily proscribe the use of certain artificial means destined solely either to the facilitating of the natural act or to ensuring that the natural act normally performed achieves its proper end."[53] If the technical means facilitates the conjugal act or helps it to reach its natural objectives, it can be morally acceptable. If, on the other hand, the procedure were to replace the conjugal act, it is morally illicit.

Artificial insemination as a substitute for the conjugal act is prohibited by reason of the voluntarily achieved dissociation of the two meanings of the conjugal act. Masturbation, through which the sperm is normally obtained, is another sign of this dissociation: Even when it is done for the purpose of procreation, the act remains deprived of its ultimate meaning: "It lacks the sexual relationship called for by the moral order, namely the relationship which realizes 'the full sense of mutual self-giving and human procreation in the context of true love.'"[54]

7. *What moral criterion can be proposed with regard to medical intervention in human procreation?* The medical act must be evaluated not only with reference to its technical dimension, but also and above all in relation to its goal, which is the good of persons and their bodily and psychological health. The moral criteria for medical intervention in procreation are deduced from the dignity of human persons, of their sexuality and of their origin.

Medicine which seeks to be ordered to the integral good of the person must respect the specifically human values of sexuality.[55] The doctor is at the service of persons and of human procreation. He does not have the authority to dispose of them or to decide their fate. A medical intervention respects the dignity of persons when it seeks to assist the conjugal act either in order to facilitate its performance or in order to enable it to achieve its objective once it has been normally performed.[56]

On the other hand, it sometimes happens that a medical procedure technologically replaces the conjugal act in order to obtain a procreation which is neither its result nor its fruit. In this case the medical act is not, as it should be, at the service of conjugal union, but rather appropriates to itself the procreative function and thus contradicts the dignity and the inalienable rights of the spouses and of the child to be born.

The humanization of medicine, which is insisted upon today by everyone, requires respect for the integral dignity of the human person first of all in the act and at the moment in which the spouses transmit life to a new person. It is only logical therefore to address an urgent appeal to Catholic doctors and scientists that they bear exemplary witness to the respect due to the human embryo and to the dignity of procreation. The medial and nursing staff of Catholic hospitals and clinics are in a special way urged to do the moral obligations which they have assumed, frequently also, as part of their contract. Those who are in charge of Catholic hospitals and clinics and who are often Religious will take special care to safeguard and promote a diligent observance of the moral norms recalled in the present Instruction.

8. *The suffering caused by infertility in marriage.* The suffering of spouses who cannot have children or who are afraid of bringing a handicapped child into the world is a suffering that everyone must understand and properly evaluate.

On the part of the spouses, the desire for a child is natural: It expresses the vocation to fatherhood and motherhood inscribed in conjugal love. This desire can be even stronger if the couple is affected by sterility which appears incurable. Nevertheless, marriage does not confer upon the spouses the right to have a child, but only the right to perform those natural acts which are per se ordered to procreation.[57]

A true and proper right to a child would be contrary to the child's dignity and nature. The child is not an object to which one has a right nor can he be considered as an object of ownership: Rather a child is a gift, "the supreme gift" and the most gratuitous gift of marriage, and is a living testimony of the mutual giving of his parents. For this reason, the child has the right, as already mentioned, to be the fruit of the specific act of the conjugal love of his parents; and he also has the right to be respected as a person from the moment of his conception. Nevertheless, whatever its cause or prognosis, sterility is certainly a difficult trial. The community of believers is called to shed light upon and support the suffering of those who are unable to fulfill their legitimate aspiration to motherhood and fatherhood. Spouses who find themselves in this sad situation are called to find in it an opportunity for sharing in a particular way in the Lord's cross, the source of spiritual fruitfulness. Sterile couples must not forget that "even when procreation is not possible, conjugal life does not for this reason lose its value. Physical sterility in fact can be for spouses the occasion for other important services to the life of the human person, for example, adoption, various forms of educational work and assistance to other families and to poor or handicapped children."[58]

Many researchers are engaged in the fight against sterility. While fully safeguarding the dignity of human procreation, some have achieved results which previously seemed unattainable. Scientists therefore are to be encouraged to continue their research with the aim of preventing the causes of sterility and of being able to remedy them so that sterile couples will be able to procreate in full respect for their own personal dignity and that of the child to be born.

III. MORAL AND CIVIL LAW

The Values and Moral Obligations that Civil Legislation Must Respect and Sanction in this Matter

The inviolable right to life of every innocent human individual and the rights of the family and of the institution of marriage constitute fundamental moral values because they concern the natural condition and integral vocation of the human person; at the same time they are constitutive elements of civil society and its order. For this reason the new technological possibilities which have opened up in the field of biomedicine require the intervention of the political authorities and of the legislator, since an uncontrolled application of such techniques could lead to unforeseeable and damaging consequences for civil society. Recourse to the conscience of each individual and to the self-regulation of researchers cannot be sufficient for ensuring respect for personal rights and public order. If the legislator responsible for the common good were not watchful, he could be deprived of his prerogatives by researchers claiming to govern humanity in the name of the biological discoveries and the alleged "improvement" processes which they would draw from those discoveries. "Eugenism" and forms of discrimination between human beings could come to be legitimized: This would constitute an act of violence and a serious offense to the equality, dignity and fundamental rights of the human person.

The intervention of the public authority must be inspired by the rational principles which regulate the relationships between civil law and moral law. The task of the civil law is to ensure the common good of people through the recognition of and the defense of fundamental rights and through the promotion of peace and of public morality.[59] In no sphere of life can the civil law take the place of conscience or dictate norms concerning things which are outside its competence. It must sometimes tolerate, for the sake of public order, things which it cannot forbid without a great evil resulting. However, the inalienable rights of the person must be recognized and respected by civil society and the political authority. These human rights depend neither on single individuals or on parents; nor do they represent a concession made by society and the state: They pertain to human nature and are inherent in the person by virtue of the creative act from which the person took his or her origin.

Among such fundamental rights one should mention in this regard:

a) every human being's right to life and physical integrity from the moment of conception until death;

b) the rights of the family and of marriage as an institution and, in this area, the child's right to be conceived, brought into the world and brought up by his parents. To each of these two themes it is necessary here to give some further consideration.

In various States (Nations) certain laws have authorized the direct suppression of innocents: The moment a positive law deprives a category of human beings of the protection which civil legislation must accord them, the state is denying the equality of all before the law. When the state does not place its power at the service of the rights of each citizen, and in particular of the more vulnerable, the very foundations of a state based on law are undermined. The political authority consequently cannot give approval to the calling of human beings into existence through procedures which would expose them to those very grave risks noted previously. The possible recognition by positive law and the political authorities of techniques of artificial transmission of life and the experimentation connected with it would widen the breach already opened by the legalization of abortion.

As a consequence of respect and protection which must be ensured for the unborn child from the moment of his conception, the law must provide appropriate penal sanctions for every deliberate violation of the child's rights. The law cannot tolerate—indeed it must expressly forbid—that human beings, even at the embryonic stage, should be treated as objects of experimentation, be mutilated or destroyed with the excuse that they are superfluous or incapable of developing normally.

The political authority is bound to guarantee to the institution of the family, upon which society is based, the juridical protection to which it has a right. From the very fact that it is at the service of people, the political authority must also be at the service of the family. Civil law cannot grant approval to techniques of artificial procreation which, for the benefit of third parties (doctors, biologists, economic or governmental powers), take away what is a right inherent in the relationship between spouses; and therefore civil law cannot legalize the donation of gametes between persons who are not legitimately united in marriage.

Legislation must also prohibit, by virtue of the support which is due to the family, embryo banks, post-mortem insemination and "surrogate motherhood."

It is part of the duty of the public authority to ensure that the civil law is regulated according to the fundamental norms of the moral law in matters concerning human rights, human life and the institution of the family. Politicians must commit themselves, through their interventions upon public opinion, to securing in society the widest possible consensus on such essential points and to consolidating this consensus wherever it risks being weakened or is in danger of collapse.

In many countries the legalization of abortion and juridical tolerance of unmarried couples makes it more difficult to secure respect for the fundamental rights recalled by this Instruction. It is to be hoped that states will not become responsible for aggravating these socially damaging situations of injustice. It is rather to be hoped that nations and states will realize all the cultural, ideological and political implications connected with the techniques of artificial procreation and will find the wisdom and courage necessary for issuing laws which are more just and more respectful of human life and the institution of the family.

The civil legislation of many states confers an undue legitimation upon certain practices in the eyes of many today; it is seen to be incapable of guaranteeing that morality which is in conformity with the natural exigencies of the human person and with the "unwritten laws" etched by the Creator upon the human heart. All men of good will must commit themselves, particularly within their professional field and in the exercise of their civil rights, to ensuring the reform of morally unacceptable civil laws and the correction of illicit practices. In addition, "conscientious objection" vis-à-vis such laws must be supported and recognized. A movement of passive resistance to the legitimation of practices contrary to human life and dignity is beginning to make an ever sharper impression upon the moral conscience of many, especially among specialists in the biomedical sciences.

Conclusion

The spread of technologies of intervention in the processes of human procreation raises very serious moral problems in relation to the respect due to the human being from the moment of conception, to the dignity of the person, of his or her sexuality and of the transmission of life.

With this Instruction the congregation for the Doctrine of the Faith, in fulfilling its responsibility to promote and defend the Church's teaching in so serious a matter, addresses a new and heartfelt invitation to all those who, by reason of their role and their commitment, can exercise a positive influence and ensure that in the family and in society due respect is accorded to life and love. It addresses this invitation to those responsible for the formation of consciences and of public opinion, to scientists and medical professionals, to jurists and politicians. It hopes that all will understand the incompatibility between recognition of the dignity of the human person and contempt for life and love, between faith in the living God and the claim to decide arbitrarily the origin and fate of a human being.

In particular, the Congregation for the Doctrine of Faith addresses an invitation with confidence and encouragement to theologians, and accessible to the faithful the contents of the teaching of the Church's Magisterium in the light of a valid anthropology in the matter of sexuality and marriage and in the context of the necessary interdisciplinary approach. Thus they will make it possible to understand ever more clearly the reasons for and the validity of this teaching. By defending man against the excesses of his own power, the Church of God reminds him of the reasons for his true nobility; only in this way can the possibility of living and loving with that dignity and liberty which derive from respect for the truth be ensured for the men and women of tomorrow. The precise indications which are offered in the present Instruction therefore are not meant to halt the effort of reflection, but rather to give it a renewed impulse in unrenounceable fidelity to the teaching of the Church.

In light of the truth about the gift of human life and in the light of the moral principles which flow from that truth, everyone is invited to act in the area of responsibility proper to each and, like the Good Samaritan, to recognize as a neighbor even the littlest among the children of men (cf. Luke 10:29-37). Here Christ's words find a new and particular echo: "What you do to one of the least of my brethren, you do unto me" (Matt. 25:40).

During an audience granted to the undersigned prefect after the plenary session of the Congregation for the Doctrine of the Faith, the Supreme Pontiff, John Paul II, approved this Instruction and ordered it to be published.

Given at Rome, from the Congregation for the Doctrine of Faith, February 22, 1987, the Feast of the Chair of St. Peter, the Apostle.

Cardinal Joseph Ratzinger,
Prefect

Archbishop Alberto Bovone,
Secretary

Appendix B

A Christ-Centered Approach to Infertility

When it comes to bearing a child, in whom will we place our highest trust—in God or modern medicine? For Christians, prayer and discernment concerning God's leading and timing in this area of life is more valuable than automatic reliance upon physicians who perform costly invasive treatments.

"We live in an age when science has become God and technology is the Holy Spirit," says childbirth educator Lynn Baptisti Richards. "We should perhaps have coins upon which are stamped, 'In Technology We Trust.'"[1]

But consider what the Old Testament proverb says:

> Trust in the LORD with all your heart
>   and lean not on your own understanding;
> In all your ways acknowledge him,
>   and he will make your paths straight.
> Do not be wise in your own eyes;
>   fear the LORD and shun evil.
> This will bring health to your body
>   and nourishment to your bones.
>
> PROVERBS 3:5-8

The Bible contains numerous stories of infertile women—Sarah, Rebekah, Rachel, Hannah, a Shunammite woman, Samson's mother and Elizabeth—who were provided with children due to God's direct intervention in their lives. [See the stories of Sarah (Genesis 11:30; 16:1—17:22; 21:1-20); Rebekah (Genesis 25:21); Rachel (Genesis 29:31—30:24); Samson's mother (Judges 13:1-24); Hannah (1 Samuel

1:1—2:11); the Shunammite woman (2 Kings 4:8-37); and Elizabeth (Luke 1:1-23).] In each of these stories, infertility plays an important role in the overall context of history.

When people failed to trust God to satisfy their desire for a child, family turmoil soon followed (Genesis 16:1-16 and 21:8-20; Genesis 30:1-21 and 37:1-36). Sarah's command that a substitute be used to bypass her infertility resulted in the spiritual bondage of an entire nation (Galatians 4:21-31). Rachel's intense desire for a second pregnancy ended in death (Genesis 35:16-19). The Bible's unfavorable portrayal of surrogacy provides a strong warning to steer clear of similar arrangements today. Artificial insemination by donor, third-party (surrogacy) pregnancy contracts, egg donation, and surrogate embryo transfer, for example, all utilize the reproductive potential and genetic heritage of someone outside the marriage covenant to produce offspring.

John T. Noonan gives the solution to this problem when he states that "to avoid reaching that condition of society where . . . breeding of human beings as objects becomes routine, the Christian insistence that procreation is indissolubly linked to conjugal love is the first and most significant safeguard."[2]

In contrast to Sarah and Rachel, Hannah's story presents an entirely different picture of a woman coping with the hidden despair of infertility:

> *In bitterness of soul Hannah wept much and prayed to the LORD. And she made a vow, saying, "O LORD Almighty, if you will only look upon your servant's misery and remember me, and not forget your servant but give her a son, then I will give him to the LORD for all the days of his life, and no razor will ever be used on his head."*
>
> *As she kept praying to the LORD, Eli observed her mouth. Hannah was praying in her heart, and her lips were moving but her voice was not heard. Eli thought she was drunk and said to her, "How long will you keep on getting drunk? Get rid of your wine."*
>
> *"Not so, my lord," Hannah replied, "I am a woman who is deeply troubled. I have not been drinking wine or beer; I was pouring out*

*my soul to the LORD. Do not take your servant for a wicked woman;
I have been praying here out of my great anguish and grief."*

*Eli answered, "Go in peace, and may the God of Israel grant you
what you have asked of him."*

*She said, "May your servant find favor in your eyes." Then she
went her way and ate something, and her face was no longer
downcast.*

1 SAMUEL 1:10-18

Hannah's prolonged childlessness brought her to a place of complete brokenness and humility before God. Rather than seeking to bear a child through using someone else, she poured out her anguish in prayer and fasting. She trusted God instead of devising her own solutions to her despair. God met Hannah at her point of need and provided her with a child she named Samuel. In response, Hannah wisely proclaimed, "The LORD brings death and makes alive; he brings down to the grave and raises up. . . . It is not by strength that one prevails" (1 Samuel 2:6, 9).

As many as one in five infertile couples receive no explanation for their condition by their physicians. Rather than viewing this situation as a dead-end diagnosis, however, couples might seize this new opportunity to deepen their faith and develop trust in God.

For some, this will mean rescuing children from abortion or abandonment through adoption as a courageous alternative to advanced reproductive technologies. For others, it may mean greater freedom to serve Christ in full-time ministry. For still others, it means God's direct, sovereign intervention will be provided according to the Lord's purposes and timing. The births of children to infertile women in the Bible are a powerful reminder of our Creator's role in procreation. *Such miracles still happen today.* Consider these examples:

- Linda and Bill, both personal friends of my family, conceived a child after a fourteen-year experience with infertility. They had long since given up "trying" to get pregnant, having reached the limit to what medicine could do for them years ago. There is no scientific explanation whatsoever for the birth of their son, Zachary. He was solely an answer to prayer.

- Josie's three babies were delivered by cesarean section, and her physician warned her that a fourth pregnancy might cause her uterus to rupture. Consequently, he recommended that she have her tubes tied while undergoing the surgical delivery of her third child. Some time later, however, Josie realized that she had gone ahead with the sterilization without really praying about it. She decided to pray and ask the Lord to reopen her womb if the tubal ligation had not been His will. The next month Josie was pregnant. When the physician performed her fourth cesarean nine months later, he was amazed to find that *a third fallopian tube* had grown from Josie's uterus! *Her original oviducts were still tightly sealed.* The ob/gyn could offer no medical reason for this phenomenon. Josie's fourth daughter is now in her teens.

- Karen was infertile for six years before she conceived her first child, and then she miscarried her second baby sixteen weeks later. Several years went by, leading Karen to start a group for infertile couples at her small church. Participants committed themselves to prayer and Bible study as well as to providing mutual support to one another. Some relied on natural means to promote fertility, while others chose medical treatment. Within just a few years, all six had borne children.

- Bev and Randy became parents in direct answer to their prayers for a child. Unable to conceive due to chemotherapy treatments for cancer, Bev continued to believe God wanted her to become a mother. Eventually, she was led to a single woman looking for a Christian couple to adopt her baby. Bev and Randy turned out to be the couple God had in mind, and they brought Joseph home just before Christmas. They have found great joy in taking him into their home to share the love they have long been waiting to give a child.

For infertile couples trying to find their way through the wilderness of today's ARTs, it may also mean finding a path to parenthood that bypasses the rocky road of high-risk, low-yield techniques and treatments. If you are facing a diagnosis of infertility, the following section of this Appendix may be particularly helpful to you.

There are five basic questions that will be useful for you to consider before entering today's complex maze of infertility diagnosis and treatment. Whether you are just thinking about scheduling an appointment with a physician or are currently in the care of a reproductive health specialist, prayerfully discussing your replies to these questions may enable you to avoid getting lost along the way.

1. Is prolonged medical treatment worth the pain, expense and disruption to our lives?

2. Might adoption or remaining childless be what the Lord would have for our lives right now?

3. Would treatment be so expensive that our financial stewardship might be jeopardized?

4. Are there any reproductive technologies I should avoid and why?

5. If it isn't time to stop treatment now, when would it be?

There are no easy answers to the pain and anguish infertility causes in a couple's life. It can be a life crisis more chronically devastating than any other, producing a wide range of emotions over a period of time—from anger to despair to a sense of hopelessness and overwhelming fatigue. These suggestions may help to ease the pain a little, as well as enable you to move through this time with greater understanding and discernment.

If you are having difficulty becoming pregnant, take time to assess your lifestyle and learn how to observe signs of fertility before resorting to medical therapy—if there are no unusual symptoms of reproductive disease or disability. Stress, diet, weight, age, exercise, and a woman's current health status all contribute to her ability to carry a baby. In addition, it is important to remember that many women have at least one or two anovulatory cycles per year (cycles in which menstruation occurs, but not ovulation) and that the average length of time it takes to conceive is eight months.

Because infertility diagnosis and treatment often involve expensive procedures without guarantees of success, it is essential to proceed carefully when selecting a health-care provider or making decisions about infertility therapy. An excellent resource covering consumer issues in infertility treatment is *Infertility: Medical and Social Choices*, available from the U.S. Government Printing Office.

The selection of a physician is one of the most important health-care decisions an infertile couple seeking medical treatment will ever make, so it is essential to shop carefully. I cannot emphasize strongly enough how important this is. Become better informed about health-care services. Don't rely solely on friends for recommendations; get references from at least four or five different consumer-oriented services and life-affirming groups such as your local crisis pregnancy center.

Join or start a Christ-centered support group for infertile couples. Only those who are experiencing a similar situation can truly understand what you are going through. Secular organizations can only go so far in ministering to hurting hearts, and yet many churches have been slow to respond to the anguish of infertile couples. Providing appropriate avenues to express this pain and grief with other believers within the body of Christ is vital.

Explore the alternative of adoption. If a child needs a home, adoption is a redemptive act that mirrors God's willingness to accept us as Christ's coheirs in His kingdom. It is not just an alternative method of having children, but a way of responding to a very real need—the need of a baby or child who might have been aborted or abandoned to know what it means to be unconditionally loved and accepted.

Prayerfully consider adopting a child of a different ethnic background or physical/mental capability than yourselves. While it has become increasingly difficult since the legalization of abortion to adopt a "perfect" or genetically similar child, special-needs children in the United States account for about 60 percent of those waiting to be adopted. Only about one-third of the approximately 36,000 available special-needs kids will be taken in any given year.

"With the great scarcity of babies for adoption now, adoptive parents are looking for children of different racial color, children of ethnic backgrounds far different from their own, and yes, even handicapped children, some of whose handicaps are staggering as one contemplates the special care and love that will be necessary to see the adoptive process through to the end," says former Surgeon General C. Everett Koop. "It is an example of Christian love, of Christian fortitude, and of the kind of social action by Christians that we talk about more than we see."

Above all, be encouraged! *God hears your prayers and knows your heart. The desire to become parents honors God. If you are willing to trust Him to control and direct this important area of your life, His grace will sustain you in remarkable and unpredictable ways.*

You don't have to turn to extreme techniques and expensive technologies to bear beautiful fruit for the Lord through ministry to your family and to the world. The Author of life hears the cry of all who diligently seek Him (Hebrews 4:14-16). Count on this: God's love never fails.

> *Our help is in the name of the* LORD,
> *Who made heaven and earth.*
>
> PSALM 124:8 NASB

NOTES

PREFACE

1 L. A. Kirkendall and M. E. Perry, "The Transition from Sex to Sensuality and Intimacy," in L. A. Kirkendall and A. E. Gravatt, eds., *Marriage and Family in the Year 2020* (New York: Prometheus, 1984), 161.

2 M. McLuhan and G. Leonard, "The future of sex," *Look*, July 25, 1967, 56-63. Italics mine.

3 Kirkendall and Gravatt, op. cit., 177.

INTRODUCTION

1 Quoted in L. Campbell, "Advances with embryos leave laws far behind," *Chicago Tribune*, April 8, 1992, C1.

2 Genesis 49:25.

ONE: LAB-ORIENTED CONCEPTIONS AND *MIS*-CONCEPTIONS

1 J. A. Robertson, *Children of Choice: Freedom and the New Reproductive Technologies* (Princeton, NJ: Princeton University Press, 1994), 5.

2 Editorial, "What comes after fertilization?" *Nature*, February 15, 1969, 613.

3 R. T. Francoeur, *Utopian Motherhood: New Trends in Human Reproduction* (Garden City, NY: Doubleday, 1970), 113.

4 For example, see: L. Shettles, "Observations on human follicular and tubal ova," *American Journal of Obstetrics and Gynecology*, 1953, 66(2): 235-247; L. Shettles, "A morula stage of human ova developed in vitro," *Fertility and Sterility*, 1955, 6(4): 287-289; L. Shettles, "Corona radiata and zona pellucida of living human ova," *Fertility and Sterility*, 1958, 9(2): 167-170; L. Mastroianni and C. Noriega, "Observations on human ova and the fertilization process," *American Journal of Obstetrics and Gynecology*, 1970, 107(5): 682-690; J. F. Kennedy and R. P. Donahue, "Human oocytes: maturation in chemically defined media," **Science** 164 (June 13, 1969): 1292-1293; P. Liedholm, P. Sundstrom, and H. Wramsky, "A model for experimental studies on human egg transfer," *Archives of Andrology*, 1980, 5(1): 92.

5 L. McLaughlin, *The Pill, John Rock and the Church* (Boston: Little, Brown and Company, 1982); A. T. Hertig, "A fifteen-year search for first-stage human ova," *Journal of the American Medical Association*, January 20, 1989, 434-435; R. Edwards and P. Steptoe, *A Matter of Life* (New York: William Morrow, 1980).

6 McLaughlin, op. cit., 41.

7 Hertig, op. cit., 434.

8 Ibid.

9 McLaughlin, op. cit., 63-64.

10 Hertig, op. cit., 435.

11 McLaughlin, op. cit., 64.

12 J. C. Doyle, "Unnecessary ovariectomies," *Journal of the American Medical Association*, March 29, 1952, 1105-1111.

13   Ibid., 1111.

14   Ibid., 1105.

15   Hertig, op. cit., 434; McLaughlin, op. cit., 68.

16   Hertig, op. cit., 435.

17   J. Rock and A. T. Hertig, "Some aspects of early human development," *American Journal of Obstetrics and Gynecology* 44 (1942): 973-983.

18   Hertig, op. cit., 435.

19   Ibid., 434.

20   J. Rock and M. F. Menkin, "In vitro fertilization and cleavage of human ovarian eggs," *Science*, August 4, 1944, 105.

21   McLaughlin, op. cit., 78.

22   Rock and Menkin, op. cit; M. F. Menkin and J. Rock, "In vitro fertilization and cleavage of human ovarian eggs," *American Journal of Obstetrics and Gynecology* 55 (March 1948): 440-454.

23   Ibid.

24   R. G. Edwards, B. D. Bavister, and P. C. Steptoe, "Early stages of fertilization in vitro of human oocytes matured in vitro," *Nature*, February 15, 1969, 632-635.

25   R. G. Edwards and P. C. Steptoe, *A Matter of Life* (New York: William Morrow, 1980), 42-43.

26   R. G. Edwards, "Maturation in vitro of mouse, sheep, cow, pig, rhesus monkey and human ovarian oocytes," *Nature*, October 23, 1965, 349-351; R. G. Edwards, "Maturation in vitro of human ovarian oocytes," *The Lancet*, November 6, 1965, 926-929.

27   Ibid., 349-350.

28   Edwards and Steptoe, *A Matter of Life*, 57.

29   R. G. Edwards, "Chromosomal abnormalities in human embryos," *Nature*, May 26, 1983, 283; R. R. Angell et al., "Chromosome abnormalities in human embryos after *in vitro* fertilization," *Nature*, May 26, 1983, 336-338; J. L. Watt et al., "Trisomy 1 in an eight cell human pre-embryo," *Journal of Medical Genetics* 24 (1987): 60-64; G. Vines, "New insight into early embryos," *New Scientist*, July 9, 1987, 22-23.

30   A. McLaren, "Can we diagnose genetic disease in pre-embryos?" *New Scientist*, December 10, 1987, 44-47; K. Johnston, "Sex of new embryos known," *Nature*, June 18, 1987, 547.

31   R. G. Edwards, "Mammalian eggs in the laboratory," *Scientific American* 215 (August 1966): 81.

32   R. G. Edwards, B. D. Bavister, and P. C. Steptoe, "Early stages of fertilization *in vitro* of human oocytes matured *in vitro*," *Nature*, February 15, 1969, 632.

33   Edwards and Steptoe, *A Matter of Life*, 186-187.

34   Ibid., 81.

35   Ibid., 82.

36   See Edwards's and Bavister's article and the accompanying editorial in *Nature*, February 15, 1969, 613, 632-635.

37   Before admission to a Catholic hospital for a diagnostic laparoscopy, I asked what would be done with my ovary or ovaries if surgery was deemed absolutely necessary. They said that ovaries removed from women there are buried, I presume out of respect for

women's reproductive dignity and the sanctity of human life. Nevertheless, I decided to include my understanding of this policy on the consent form for my surgery. For any woman undergoing surgery today in which ovarian tissue might be removed, I strongly recommend including a statement such as this: "It is my understanding that it is the policy of this hospital to bury surgically removed ovaries. In the event that an ovariectomy is necessary, I request that all ovarian tissue taken from me by this method be buried without prior oocyte removal." My gynecologist, who is a woman, understood my request. If the hospital had not had this policy, I would have made my own arrangements for the safe disposal of my ova.

TWO: SEX IN A DISH?

1   D. Bonhoeffer, *Ethics* (New York: Macmillan, 1955, 1975), 148.

2   D. Del Zio, "I was cheated of my test-tube baby," *Good Housekeeping*, March 1979, 203.

3   Ibid., 135.

4   Ibid., 200.

5   Ibid.

6   Ibid.

7   Ibid.

8   L. Shettles, "Observations on human follicular and tubal ova," *American Journal of Obstetrics and Gynecology*, 1953, 66(2): 235-247; L. Shettles, "A morula stage of human ova developed in vitro," *Fertility and Sterility*, 1955, 6(4): 287-289; L. Shettles, "Corona radiata and zona pellucida of living human ova," *Fertility and Sterility*, 1958, 9(2): 167-170.

9   Del Zio, op. cit., 200.

10   Ibid., 202.

11   U.S. Congress, Office of Technology Assessment, *Infertility: Medical and Social Choices* (Washington, DC: U.S. Government Printing Office, 1988), 36.

12   L. R. Kass, "Babies by in vitro fertilization: unethical experiments on the unborn?" *New England Journal of Medicine*, November 18, 1971, 1176-1178.

13   R. Edwards and P. Steptoe, *A Matter of Life* (New York: William Morrow, 1980), 87.

14   Ibid., 88.

15   Cited in Kass, op. cit., 1178.

16   Edwards and Steptoe, op. cit., 118.

17   Ibid., 90.

18   Ibid.

19   Ibid., 90-91.

20   Ibid., 96-97.

21   Edwards is quite vague about the exact dates of IVF experiments in his book. However, in *A Matter of Life*, he says on page 89 that he and Bavister fertilized the first human eggs "last October." He later points out this was during the year before *Nature* published his paper about the experiment (in March 1969). This places the year in which the first human IVF took place as 1968.

22   Ibid., 92.

23   Ibid., 118.

24   Again Edwards avoids giving out exact dates, but one can put the pieces together by other events he provides dates for in his book.

25   R. G. Edwards and R. E. Fowler, "Human embryos in the laboratory," *Scientific American* 223 (1970): 50.

26   Ibid., 49.

27   The Nuremberg Military Tribunal's decision in the case of *United States v. Karl Brandt et al.* provides a set of clear guidelines for medical experimentation in what is known as the *Nuremberg Code*. In the wake of Nazi war crimes committed during World War II, the Tribunal declared that if treatments of an experimental nature are provided by physicians, the voluntary consent of the subject participating in the research is absolutely essential.
      This means that the person involved should have legal capacity to give consent; should be so situated as to be able to exercise free power of choice, without the intervention of any element of force, fraud, deceit, duress, over-reaching, or other ulterior form of constraint or coercion; and should have sufficient knowledge and comprehension of the elements of the subject matter involved as to enable him/her to make an understanding and enlightened decision. This latter element requires that before the acceptance of an affirmative decision by the experimental subject there should be made known to him/her the nature, duration, and purpose of the experiment; the method and means by which it is to be conducted; all inconveniences and hazards reasonably to be expected; and the effects upon his/her health or person which may possibly come from his/her participation in the experiment. . . .
      The experiment should be so designed and based on the results of animal experimentation and a knowledge of the natural history of the disease or other problem (in this case, IVF) under study that the anticipated results will justify the performance of the experiment. (From D. Ch. Overduin and J. I. Fleming, *Life in a Test Tube* [Adelaide, South Australia: Lutheran Publishing House, 1982], 226-227.)
      The anticipated results could not possibly have been known by Doris Del Zio and Dr. Steptoe's patients: There had been no trials of IVF in higher animals preceding IVF experiments in humans. Apparently, the researchers had no idea how effective or successful IVF would be.

28   For background information, see Committee on Small Business, *Consumer Protection Issues Involving In Vitro Fertilization Clinics* (Washington, DC: U.S. Government Printing Office, 1989).

29   Committee on Small Business, op. cit., 39.

30   Ibid.

31   Medical Research International and the American Fertility Society Special Interest Group, "In vitro fertilization/embryo transfer in the United States: 1985 and 1986 results from the national IVF/ET registry," *Fertility and Sterility* 49 (February 1988): 212-215.

32   Committee on Small Business, *Consumer Protection Issues Involving In Vitro Fertilization Clinics* (Washington, DC: U.S. Government Printing Office, 1988), 11, 17. For documentation of the explosion of ART in America, see: J. D. Biggers, "In vitro fertilization and embryo transfer in human beings," *New England Journal of Medicine*, February 5, 1981, 336-341; A. Clark et al., "Social and reproductive characteristics of the first 100 couples treated by in-vitro fertilization programme at national women's hospital, Auckland," *New Zealand Medical Journal*, June 24, 1987, 380-382; "Success rates for IVF and GIFT," *Contemporary OB/GYN*, May 1988, 89-106; J. E. Buster and M. V. Sauer,

"Nonsurgical donor ovum transfer: new option for infertile couples," *Contemporary OB/GYN,* August 1986, 39-49; I. Craft et al., "Analysis of 1071 gift procedures—the case for a flexible approach to treatment," *The Lancet,* May 16, 1988, 1094-1097; I. Craft et al., "Successful pregnancies from the transfer of pronucleate embryos in an outpatient in vitro fertilization program," *Fertility and Sterility* 44 (August 1985): 181-184; A. H. DeCherney and G. Lavy, "Oocyte recovery methods in in-vitro fertilization," *Clinical Obstetrics and Gynecology* 29 (March 1986): 171-179; J. Deschacht et al., "In vitro fertilization with husband and donor sperm in patients with previous fertilization failures using husband's sperm," *Human Reproduction* 3 (January 1988): 105-108; K. S. Edwards, "Reproduction technology: a guide to what's available in Ohio," *OHIO Medicine* March 1988, 183-190, 193; R. Frydman et al., "A new approach to follicular stimulation for in vitro fertilization: programmed oocyte retrieval," *Fertility and Sterility* 46 (October 1986): 657-659; R. Frydman et al., "An obstetric assessment of the first 100 births from the in vitro fertilization program at Clamart, France," *American Journal of Obstetrics and Gynecology* 154 (March 1986): 550-555; R. Frydman et al., "Programmed oocyte retrieval during routine laparoscopy and embryo cryopreservation for later transfer," *American Journal of Obstetrics and Gynecology* 155 (July 1986): 112-117; H. Jones et al., "An analysis of the obstetric outcome of 125 consecutive pregnancies conceived in vitro and resulting in 100 deliveries," *American Journal of Obstetrics and Gynecology* 154 (April 1986): 848-854; H. Jones, "The impact of in vitro fertilization on the practice of gynecology and obstetrics," *International Journal of Fertility* 31 (1986): 99-111; H. Jones et al., "The efficiency of human reproduction after in vitro fertilization and embryo transfer," *Fertility and Sterility* 49 (April 1988): 649-653; H. Jones et al., "The program for in vitro fertilization at Norfolk," *Fertility and Sterility* 38 (July 1982): 14-20; G. B. Kolata, "In vitro fertilization goes commercial," *Science* 221 (September 1983): 1160-1161; J. Leeton et al., "The technique for embryo transfer," *Fertility and Sterility* 38 (August 1982): 156-161; "100 test-tube babies gather in Baltimore," *Lincoln Journal,* September 12, 1988, A6; "In vitro clinics span globe; spawn new treatments," *Lincoln Sunday Journal-Star,* July 24, 1988, 1A, 6A; R. P. Marrs, "Human in-vitro fertilization," *Clinical Obstetrics and Gynecology* 29 (March 1986): 117; R. P. Marrs, "Laboratory conditions for human in-vitro fertilization procedures," *Clinical Obstetrics and Gynecology* 29 (March 1986): 180-189; Medical Research International and the American Fertility Society Special Interest Group, "In vitro fertilization/embryo transfer in the United States: 1985 and 1986, results from the national IVF/ET registry," *Fertility and Sterility* 49 (February 1988): 212-215; D. R. Meldrum et al., "Evolution of a highly successful in vitro fertilization-embryo transfer program," *Fertility and Sterility* 48 (July 1987): 86-93; S. Pace-Owens, "In vitro fertilization and embryo transfer," *JOGN Nursing,* Supplement (November/December 1985): 44S-48S; C. Ranoux et al., "A new in vitro fertilization technique: intravaginal culture," *Fertility and Sterility* 49 (April 1988): 654-657; C. Ranoux et al., "Intravaginal culture and embryo transfer: a new method for the fertilization of human oocytes," *Review of French Gynecology and Obstetrics* 82 (December 1987): 741-744; J. M. Rary et. al., "Techniques of in vitro fertilization of oocytes and embryo transfer in humans," *Archives of Andrology* 5 (1980): 89-90; C. A. Raymond, "IVF registry notes more centers, more births, slightly improved odds," *Journal of the American Medical Association,* April 1, 1988, 1920-1921; V. Sharma et al., "An analysis of factors influencing the establishment of a clinical pregnancy in an ultrasound-based ambulatory in vitro fertilization clinic," *Fertility and Sterility* 49 (March 1988): 468-478; P. H. Wessels et al., "Gamete intrafallopian transfer: a treatment for long-standing infertility," *Journal of In Vitro Fertilization and Embryo Transfer* 4

(October 1987): 256-259; P. C. Wong et al., "Eighty consecutive cases of gamete intrafallopian transfer," *Human Reproduction* 3 (February 1988): 231-233; C. Wood et al., "Clinical features of eight pregnancies resulting from in vitro fertilization and embryo transfer," *Fertility and Sterility* 38 (July 1982): 22; C. Wood et al., "Factors influencing pregnancy rates following in vitro fertilization and embryo transfer," *Fertility and Sterility* 43 (1985): 245-250; J. L. Yovich et al., "Place of GIFT in infertility services," *The Lancet*, February 27, 1988, 470; J. L. Yovich et al. , "Pregnancies following pronuclear stage tubal transfer," *Fertility and Sterility* 48 (November 1987): 851-857; J. L. Yovich et al., "PROST for ovum donation," *The Lancet*, May 23, 1987, 1209-1210.

33 L. Silver, *Remaking Eden* (New York: Avon, 1997), 80.

34 Society for Assisted Reproductive Technology, "Assisted reproductive techniques in the United States and Canada: 1994 results generated from the American Society of Reproductive Medicine/Society for Assisted Reproductive Technology Registry," *Fertility and Sterility* 66 (1996): 697-705.

35 L. Gubernick, "Easier than selling soap," *Forbes*, February 9, 1987, 113-114.

36 C. A. Raymond, "In vitro fertilization enters stormy adolescence as experts debate the odds," *Journal of the American Medical Association*, January 22/29, 1988, 464.

37 M. Shearer, "Some effects of assisted reproduction on perinatal care," *Birth* 15 (1988): 131-132.

38 H. Jones et al., "What is a pregnancy? A question for programs of in vitro fertilization," *Fertility and Sterility* 40 (December 1983): 728-733; A. F. Haney, "What is efficacious infertility therapy?" *Fertility and Sterility* 48 (October 1987): 543-545; R. J. Lilford and M. E. Dalton, "Effectiveness of treatment for infertility," *British Medical Journal*, July 18, 1987, 155-156; D. Berstein et al., "Is conception in infertile couples treatment-related?" *International Journal of Fertility* 24 (1979): 65-67; J. Jarrell et al., "An in vitro fertilization and embryo transfer pilot study: treatment-dependent and treatment-independent pregnancies," *American Journal of Obstetrics and Gynecology* 154 (February 1986): 231-235; S. I. Roh et al., "In vitro fertilization and embryo transfer: treatment-dependent versus -independent pregnancies," *Fertility and Sterility* 48 (December 1987): 982-986.

39 M. M. Seibel, "In vitro fertilization success rates: a fraction of the truth," *Obstetrics & Gynecology* 72 (August 1988): 265-266; M. R. Soules, "The in vitro fertilization pregnancy rate: let's be honest with one another," *Fertility and Sterility* 43 (April 1985): 511-513. See also: A. Bonnicksen, "Some consumer aspects of in vitro fertilization and embryo transfer," *Birth* 15 (1988): 148-151; A. L. Bonnicksen and R. H. Blank, "The government and in vitro fertilization (IVF): views of IVF directors," *Fertility and Sterility* 49 (March 1988): 396-398; "Ethical dilemmas of infertility," *Contemporary OB/GYN*, March 1987.

40 Gubernick, op. cit., 113-114.

41 Committee on Small Business, op. cit., 26-27.

42 J. M. Alexander et al., "Multifetal reduction of high-order multiple pregnancy: a comparison of obstetrical outcome with non-reduced twin gestations," *Fertility and Sterility* 64 (1995): 1201-1203.

43 A. Lopata, "Concepts in human in vitro fertilization and embryo transfer," *Fertility and Sterility* 40 (September 1983): 289-301; I. Craft et al., "How many oocytes/embryos should be transferred?" *The Lancet*, July 11, 1987, 109-110.

44 A. Aberg et al., "Cardiac puncture of fetus with Hurler's disease avoiding abortion of unaffected co-twin," *The Lancet*, November 4, 1978, 990-991.

45 Ibid., 990.

46 Ibid, 991. For further reading on the implications of medically promoted eugenic abortion, see L. Alexander, "Medical science under dictatorship," *New England Journal of Medicine,* July 14, 1949, 39-47; F. Ausubel, J. Beckwith, and K. Janssen, "The politics of genetic engineering: who decides who's defective?" *Psychology Today,* June 1974, 31-41; L. Blumberg, "The right to live: disability is not a crime," *The Exceptional Parent,* December 1984, 22-24; J. Bopp, ed. *Human Life and Health Care Ethics* (Frederick, MD: University Publications of America, 1985); J. Burtchaell, *Rachel Weeping,* chapter 3 (New York: Harper & Row, 1982); L. G. Cohen, "Selective abortion and the diagnosis of fetal damage: issues and concerns," *Journal of the Association for Persons with Severe Handicaps* 11 (1986): 188-195; Department of Health and Human Services, "Services and treatment for disabled infants; interim model guidelines for health care providers to establish infant review committees," 49 *Federal Register,* no. 238, December 10, 1984, 48170-48173; L. A. Fiedler, "The tyranny of the normal," *The Hastings Center Report,* April 1984, 40-42; Foundation on Economic Trends, *Human Reproductive Technologies, Genetic Screening and Human Genetic Engineering* (Washington, DC: Foundation on Economic Trends, 1988); C. Frankel, "The specter of eugenics," *Commentary,* March 1974, 25-33; M. Johnson, "Life unworthy of life," *The Disability Rag,* January/February, 1987, 24-26; R. R. Lenke and J. Nemes, "Wrongful birth, wrongful life: the doctor between a rock and a hard place," *Obstetrics & Gynecology* 66 (November 1985): 719-722; F. Schaeffer and C. E. Koop, *Whatever Happened to the Human Race?* (Wheaton, IL: Crossway Books, 1983); G. Will, "Discretionary killing," *Newsweek,* September 20, 1976.

    For a sample of readings favoring the eugenic elimination of human beings, see: H. T. Engelhardt, "Euthanasia and children: the injury of continued existence," *Journal of Pediatrics* 83 (July 1973): 170-171; J. Fletcher, "Ethical aspects of genetic controls: designed genetic changes in man," *New England Journal of Medicine,* September 30, 1971, 776-783; B. Glass, "Science: endless horizons or golden age?" *Science,* January 8, 1971, 23-29; P. Singer, "Sanctity of life or quality of life?" *Pediatrics* 72 (July 1983): 128-129.

47 H. H. H. Kanhai et al., "Selective termination in quintuplet pregnancy during first trimester," *The Lancet,* June 21, 1986, 1447; D. F. Farquharson et al., "Management of quintuplet pregnancy by selective embryocide," *American Journal of Obstetrics and Gynecology* 158 (February 1988): 413-416; M. I. Evans et al., "Selective first trimester termination octuplet and quadruplet pregnancies: clinical and ethical issues," *Obstetrics & Gynecology* 71 (March 1988): 289-296; R. L. Berkowitz et al., "Selective reduction of multifetal pregnancies in the first trimester," *New England Journal of Medicine,* April 21, 1988, 1043-1047; R. L. Berkowitz et al., "Selective reduction of multifetal pregnancies (Reply)," *New England Journal of Medicine,* October 6, 1988, 950-951; J. M. Lorenz and J. S. Terry, "Selective reduction of multifetal pregnancies (Letter)," *New England Journal of Medicine,* October 6, 1988, 949-950; S. L. Romney, "Selective reduction of multifetal pregnancies (Letter)," *New England Journal of Medicine ,* October 6, 1988, 949; J. Shalev et al., "Selective reduction of multifetal pregnancies (Letter)," *New England Journal of Medicine,* October 6, 1988, 949; E. F. Diamond, "Selective reduction of multifetal pregnancies (Letter)," *New England Journal of Medicine,* October 6, 1988, 950; D. H. James, "Selective reduction of multifetal pregnancies (Letter)," *New England Journal of Medicine,* October 6, 1988, 950; I. Craft et al., "Multiple pregnancy, selective reduction, and flexible treatment," *The Lancet,* November 5, 1988, 1087; "Selective fetus destruction debated," *Lincoln Journal,* April 21, 1988, A5.

For additional insights on how the subject of "fetal reduction" has been presented in popular women's magazines, see: "Tell us what you think: is it wrong to terminate some fetuses during a multiple pregnancy?" *Glamour,* July 1988, 50; "This is what you thought: 57 percent say a woman should have the right to terminate some fetuses," *Glamour,* September 1988, 197; "Choices," *Woman's World,* January 3, 1989, 44-45.

48   R. Frydman et al., "Reduction of the number of embryos in a multiple pregnancy: from quintuplet to triplet," *Fertility and Sterility* 48 (August 1987): 326-327.

49   Ibid., 326.

50   Ibid., 326-327.

51   Romney, op. cit., 949.

52   B. Hilton, D. Callahan, M. Harris, P. Condliffe, and B. Berkley, *Ethical Issues in Human Genetics* (New York: Plenum Press, 1973), 19.

53   American Fertility Society Committee on Ethics, "Biomedical research and respect for the preembryo," *Fertility and Sterility* 46 (February 1988), Supplement 1: 3S-4S; American Fertility Society Committee on Ethics, "Research on preembryos: justifications and limitations," *Fertility and Sterility* 46 (September 1986), Supplement 1: 56S-57S; J. Brown, "Research on human embryos—a justification," *Journal of Medical Ethics* 12 (1986): 201-205; V. Bolton et al., "GIFT in a district hospital," *The Lancet,* January 3, 1987, 50; V. Bolton, P. Braude, and S. Moore, "Ethical bounds," *Nature,* September 29, 1988, 392; V. Bolton, P. Braude, and S. Moore, "Human gene expression first occurs between the four- and eight-cell stages of preimplantation development," *Nature,* March 31, 1988, 459-461; "When life begins: embryo research," *Current,* May 1987, 9-10; S. Dickman, "West German research agencies oppose new embryo law," *Nature,* May 7, 1987, 6; S. Dickman, "Embryo research ban causes ructions in West Germany," *Nature,* June 30, 1988, 791; S. Dickman, "International outlook for embryo research," *Nature,* June 30, 1988, 6; H. J. Evans and A. McLaren, "Unborn children (protection) bill," *Nature,* March 14, 1985, 127-128; C. B. Fehilly et al., "Cryopreservation of cleaving embryos and expanded blastocysts in the human: a comparative study," *Fertility and Sterility* 44 (November 1985): 638-644; "Research on human embryos," *The Lancet,* December 13, 1986, 1375; "Draft Legislation on infertility services and embryo research," *The Lancet,* December 5, 1987, 1343; "Human embryo research: vote for progress," *The Lancet,* December 5, 1987, 1311; S. E. Lanzendorf et al., "A preclinical evaluation of pronuclear formation of human spermatozoa into human oocytes," *Fertility and Sterility* 59 (May 1988): 835-842; B. Lassalle, J. Testart, and J. Renard, "Human embryo features that influence the success of cryopreservation with the use of 1, 2 propanediol," *Fertility and Sterility* 44 (November 1985): 64; J. L. Marx, "Embryology," *Science,* November 23, 1973, 811-814; "Britain hazards embryo research," *Nature,* December 3, 1987, 407; "More embryo research?" *Nature,* May 19, 1988, 194; "UK agonizes over embryo research," *Nature,* February 7, 1985; F. Puissant et al., "Embryo scoring as a prognostic tool in IVF treatments," *Human Reproduction* 2 (November 1987): 705-708; J. Testart et al., "Factors influencing the success rate of human embryo freezing in an in vitro fertilization and embryo transfer program," *Fertility and Sterility* 48 (July 1987): 107-112; J. Testart et al., "Human embryo viability related to freezing and thawing procedures," *American Journal of Obstetrics and Gynecology* 157 (June 1987): 168-171; J. Townsend, "Research on human embryos," *The Lancet,* January 3, 1987, 53; A. Trounson et al., "Fertilization of human oocytes by microinjection of a single spermatozoon under the zona pellucida," *Fertility and Sterility* 48 (October 1987): 637-642; A. Trounson et al., "Tripronuclear human oocytes: altered

cleavage patterns and subsequent karotypic analysis of embryos," *Biological Reproduction* 37 (September 1987): 395-401.

54 L. R. Kass, "New Beginnings in Life," in M. Hamilton, ed., *The New Genetics and the Future of Man* (Grand Rapids, MI: William B. Eerdmans, 1971), 21, 53, 54.

55 For further information on risks related to advanced reproductive technologies, see: J. Ashkenazi et al., "Abdominal complications following ultrasonically guided percutaneous transvesical collection of oocytes for in vitro fertilization," *Journal of In Vitro Fertilization and Embryo Transfer* 4 (December 1987): 316-318; M. A. Rossing et al., "Ovarian tumors in a cohort of infertile women," *New England Journal of Medicine* 331 (1994):771; A. Venn et al., "Breast and ovarian cancer incidence after infertility and in vitro fertilization," *The Lancet*, 1995, 995-1000; J. G. Schenker and D. Weinstein, "Ovarian hyperstimulation syndrome: a current survey," *Fertility and Sterility* 30 (1978): 255-268; J. Ashkenasi et al., "Multiple pregnancy after in-vitro fertilization and embryo transfer: report of a quadruplet pregnancy and delivery," *Human Reproduction* 2 (August 1987): 511-515; F. R. Batzer et al., "Multiple pregnancies with gamete intrafallopian transfer (GIFT): Complications of a New Technique," *Journal of In Vitro Fertilization and Embryo Transfer* 5 (February 1988): 35-37; J. G. Schenker et al., "Multiple pregnancies following induction of ovulation," *Fertility and Sterility* 35 (1981):105-123; G. Byrne, "Artificial insemination report prompts call for regulation," *Science*, August 19, 1988, 895; E. Chargaff, "Engineering a molecular nightmare," *Nature*, May 21, 1987, 199-200; H. B. Holmes, "In vitro fertilization: reflections on the state of the art," *Birth* 15 (September 1988): 1134-1144; R. Hubbard with W. Sanford, "New Reproductive Technologies," in *The New Our Bodies, Ourselves*, The Boston Women's Health Collective (New York: Simon & Schuster, 1984); W. R. Phipps, C. B. Benson, and P. M. McShane, "Severe thigh myositis following intramuscular progesterone injections in an in vitro fertilization patient," *Fertility and Sterility* 49 (March 1988): 536-537; F. V. Price, "The risk of high multiparity with IVF/ET," *Birth* 15 (September 1988): 157-163; J. J. Schlesselman, "How does one assess the risk of abnormalities from human in vitro fertilization?" *American Journal of Obstetrics and Gynecology*, September 1, 1979, 135-148; D. H. Smith et al., "Tubal pregnancy occurring after successful in vitro fertilization and embryo transfer," *Fertility and Sterility* 38 (July 1982): 105-106; J. L. Yovich, S. R. Turner, and A. J. Murphy, "Embryo transfer technique as a cause of ectopic pregnancies in in vitro fertilization," *Fertility and Sterility* 44 (September 1985): 318-321.

THREE: THE BY-PRODUCTS OF MANUFACTURED CONCEPTION

1 E. Chargaff, "Engineering a molecular nightmare," *Nature*, May 21, 1987, 199. Professor Chargaff's work in biochemistry during the late 1940s led to the discovery of DNA.

2 H. I. Abdalla and T. Leonard, "Cryopreserved zygote intrafallopian transfer for anonymous oocyte donation," *The Lancet*, April 9, 1988, 835; American Fertility Society Committee on Ethics, "Donor eggs in in vitro fertilization," *Fertility and Sterility* 46 (September 1986), Supplement 1: 42S-44S; American Fertility Society Committee on Ethics, "Donor sperm in in vitro fertilization," *Fertility and Sterility* 46 (September 1986), Supplement 1: 39S-41S; American Fertility Society Committee on Ethics, "Surrogate gestational mothers: women who gestate a genetically unrelated embryo," *Fertility and Sterility* 46 (September 1986), Supplement 1: 58S-61S; L. B. Andrews, "Embryo technology," *Parent's Magazine* 56 (May 1981): 63-71; L. B. Andrews, "Legal and ethical aspects of new reproductive technologies," *Clinical Obstetrics and*

Gynecology 29 (March 1986): 190-204; L. B. Andrews, *New Conceptions* (New York: Ballantine Books, 1985); L. B. Andrews, "Yours, mine and theirs," *Psychology Today,* December 1984, 20-29; G. Annas and J. F. Henahan, "Fertilization, embryo transfer procedures raise many questions," *Journal of the American Medical Association,* August 17, 1984, 877-879, 882; G. Annas, "Making babies without sex: the law and the profits," *American Journal of Public Health* 74 (December 1984): 1415-1417; G. Annas, "Redefining parenthood and protecting embryos: why we need new laws," *The Hastings Center Report,* October 1984, 50-52; G. Annas and S. Elias, "Social policy considerations in noncoital reproduction," *Journal of the American Medical Association,* January 3, 1986, 62-68; P. Bagne, "High-tech breeding," *Mother Jones* 8 (August 1983): 23-29, 35; J. E. Buster, "Survey of attitudes regarding the use of siblings for gamete donation," *Fertility and Sterility* 49 (April 1988): 721-722; J. F. Correy, "Donor oocyte pregnancy with transfer of deep-frozen embryo," *Fertility and Sterility* 49 (March 1988): 534-535; I. Craft and J. Yovich, "Implications of embryo transfer," *The Lancet,* September 22, 1979, 642-643; I. Craft and P. F. Serhal, "Ovum donation—a simplified approach," *Fertility and Sterility* 48 (August 1987): 265-269; D. J. Cuisine, "Some legal implications of embryo transfer," *The Lancet,* August 25, 1979, 407-408; M. Curie-Cohen, L. Luttrell, and S. Shapiro, "Current practice of artificial insemination by donor in the United States," *New England Journal of Medicine,* March 15, 1979, 585-590; R. Fitzhugh, "Where's poppa?" *US Magazine,* October 22, 1984, 68-69; "What are the moral rights of frozen embryos?" *Health Progress,* October 1984, 54, 62; D. A. Iddenden, H. N. Sallam, and W. P. Collins, "A prospective randomized study comparing fresh semen and cryopreserved semen for artificial insemination by donor," *International Journal of Fertility* 30 (1985): 54-56; R. P. S. Jansen, "Sperm and ova as property," *Journal of Medical Ethics* 11 (1985): 123-126; M. Johnston, "I gave birth to another woman's baby," *Redbook,* May 1984, 44 and 46; A. M. Junca et al., "Anonymous and non-anonymous oocyte donation preliminary results," *Human Reproduction* 3 (January 1988): 121-123; H. D. Krause, "Artificial conception, legislative approaches," *Family Law Quarterly* 19 (Fall 1988): 185-206; C. Krauthammer, "The ethics of human manufacture," *The New Republic,* May 4, 1987, 17-21; J. F. Leeton et al., "Donor oocyte pregnancy with transfer of deep-frozen embryo," *Fertility and Sterility* 49 (March 1988): 534-535; J. F. Leeton et al., "Successful pregnancy in an ovulating recipient following the transfer of two frozen-thawed embryos obtained from anonymously donated oocytes," *Journal of In Vitro Fertilization and Embryo Transfer* 5 (February 1988): 22-24; J. Leeton and J. Harman, "The donation of oocytes to known recipients," *Australia and New Zealand Journal of Obstetrics and Gynaecology* 27 (August 1987): 248-250; "Woman bears own grandchild," *Lincoln Journal,* October 1, 1987, 2; "Babies: no sale," *Los Angeles Times,* February 4, 1988; M. Madhevan, A. O. Trounson, and J. F. Leeton, "Successful use of human semen cryobanking for in vitro fertilization," *Fertility and Sterility* 40 (September 1983): 340-343; M. C. Michelow, "Mother-daughter in vitro fertilization triplet surrogate pregnancy," *Journal of In Vitro Fertilization and Embryo Transfer* 5 (February 1988): 31-34; H. J. Muller, "Human evolution by voluntary choice of germ plasm," *Science,* September 8, 1961, 643-649; M. Novak, "Buying & selling babies: limitations on the marketplace," *Commonweal,* July 17, 1987, 406-407; J. Salat-Baroux et al., "Pregnancies after replacement of frozen-thawed embryos in a donation program," *Fertility and Sterility* 49 (March 1988): 817-821; R. G. Seed and R. W. Seed, "Embryo adoption—technical, ethical and legal aspects," *Archives in Andrology* 5 (1980); R. Snowden and G. D. Mitchell, *Artificial Reproduction: A Social Investigation* (London: George Allen & Unwin, 1983); R. Snowden and G. D. Mitchell, *The Artificial Family: A*

Consideration of Artificial Insemination by Donor (London: George Allen & Unwin, 1981); R. C. Strickler, D. W. Keller, and J. C. Warren, "Artificial insemination with fresh donor semen," *New England Journal of Medicine*, October 23, 1975, 848-853; J. L. Yovich, "Surrogacy," *The Lancet*, June 13, 1987, 1374.

3 B. Katz Rothman, "How science is redefining parenthood," *Ms.*, July/August 1982, 154, 156.

4 G. Hanscombe, "The right to lesbian parenthood," *Journal of Medical Ethics* 9 (1983): 133-135; B. Kritchevsky, "The unmarried woman's right to artificial insemination: a call for expanded definition of family," *Harvard Women's Law Journal* 4 (1981): 1-42; Lambda Legal Defense and Education Fund, Inc., Lesbian Rights Project (San Francisco), Office of Gay and Lesbian Health Concerns (NYC Department of Health), and New York University Women's Center, *Lesbians Choosing Motherhood* (New York: Lambda Legal Defense and Education Fund, Inc., 1984); Lesbian Health Information Project, *Artificial Insemination: An Alternative Conception for the Lesbian and Gay Community* (San Francisco, CA: San Francisco Women's Centers, 1979); S. Robinson and H. F. Pizer, *Having a Baby Without a Man* (New York: Simon & Schuster/Fireside Books, 1987); S. Stern, "Lesbian insemination," *The CoEvolution Quarterly*, Summer 1980, 108-117.

5 S. Callahan, "Lovemaking and baby making," *Commonweal*, April 24, 1987, 237. See also S. Callahan, "Use of third-party donors threatens basic values," *Health Progress*, March 1987, 26-28.

6 Ibid.

7 L. R. Kass, *Toward a More Natural Science: Biology and Human Affairs* (New York: The Free Press, 1985), 225.

8 P. Ramsey, "Shall we 'reproduce'? Part II. Rejoinders and future forecast," *Journal of the American Medical Association*, June 12, 1972, 1484-1485. See also: P. Ramsey, "Shall we 'reproduce'? Part I. The medical ethics of in vitro fertilization," *Journal of the American Medical Association*, June 5, 1972, 1346-1350; P. Ramsey, *Fabricated Man* (New Haven, CN: Yale University Press, 1970).

9 R. G. Seed, R. W. Seed, and D. S. Baker, "Aspects of bovine embryo transplant directly applicable to humans—a report of over 300 procedures," *Fertility and Sterility* 28 (March 1977): 313-314.

10 R. G. Seed and R. Weiss, "Embryo adoption—technical, ethical and legal aspects," *Archives in Andrology* 5 (1980); R. G. Seed and R. W. Seed, "Artificial embryonation—human embryo transplant," *Archives in Andrology* 5 (1980): 90-91.

11 A. Taylor Fleming, "New frontiers in conception," *New York Times Magazine*, July 20, 1980, 42.

12 F. Schumer Chapman, "Going for the gold in the baby business," *Fortune*, September 17, 1984, 41. Curiously, most third-party pregnancy contracts during the same time period called for "surrogate" mothers to be paid exactly the same amount.

13 Ibid., 49.

14 Ibid., 46.

15 For an interesting discussion on SET from a lawyer's point of view, see D. J. Cuisine, "Some legal implications of embryo transfer," *The Lancet*, August 25, 1979, 407-408.

16 Seed, Seed, and Baker, op. cit.

17 Ibid.

18   G. Corea, *The Mother Machine* (New York: Harper & Row/Perennial Library, 1986), 82.

19   Ibid.

20   Fleming, op. cit.

21   Ibid.

22   Seed and Seed, op. cit.; J. E. Buster, R. W. Seed, and R. G. Seed et al., "Nonsurgical ovum transfer as a treatment in infertile women," *Journal of the American Medical Association*, March 2, 1984, 1171-1173; Corea, op. cit., 83; Fleming, op. cit.

23   J. Ellul, *The Technological Society* (New York: Alfred A. Knopf, Vintage Books Edition, 1964), 10.

24   Chapman, op. cit. Buster, Seed, and Seed et al., op. cit. See also: J. E. Buster et al., "Survey of attitudes regarding the use of siblings for gamete donation," *Fertility and Sterility* 49 (April 1988): 721-722; J. E. Buster et al., "An instrument for the recovery of preimplantation uterine ova," *Obstetrics & Gynecology* 71 (May 1988): 804-806.

25   Chapman, op. cit., 42.

26   A. Trounson and L. Mohr, "Human pregnancy following cryopreservation, thawing and transfer of an eight-cell embryo," *Nature*, October 20, 1983, 707-709; A. Trounson, "Pregnancy established in an infertile patient after transfer of a donated embryo fertilised in vitro," *British Medical Journal*, March 12, 1983, 835-838; A. Trounson et al., "Effect of growth in culture medium on the rate of mouse embryo development and viability in vitro," *Journal of In Vitro Fertilization and Embryo Transfer* 4 (October 1987): 265-268; A. Trounson, "Preservation of human eggs and embryos," *Fertility and Sterility* 46 (July 1986): 1-11; A. Trounson, A. Peura, and C. Kirby, "Ultrarapid freezing: a new low-cost and effective method of embryo cryopreservation," *Fertility and Sterility* 48 (November 1987): 843-850; A. Trounson et al., "Ultrarapid freezing of early cleavage stage human embryos and eight-cell mouse embryos," *Fertility and Sterility* 49 (May 1988): 822-826; S. Al Hassani et al., "Cryopreservation of human oocytes," *Human Repoduction* 2 (November 1987): 695-700.

27   J. E. Buster and M. V. Sauer, "Nonsurgical donor ovum transfer: new option for infertile couples," *Contemporary OB/GYN*, August 1986, 39-49; Buster, Seed, and Seed et al., op. cit., 1172.

28   Corea, op. cit., 85.

29   Buster, Seed, and Seed et al., op. cit., 1171.

30   Corea, op. cit., 85; "Ovum donor transfer may see wide use in treating infertility," *Ob/Gyn News*, December 1, 1983, 1.

31   Corea, op. cit., 85.

32   Ibid., 86.

33   Buster, Seed, and Seed et al., op. cit., 1171.

34   J. E. Buster, R. W. Seed, and R. G. Seed et al., "Nonsurgical ovum transfer of in vivo fertilized donated ova to five infertile women: report of two pregnancies," *The Lancet*, July 23, 1983, 223-224.

35   Corea, op. cit., 80.

36   Sauer and Buster et al., op. cit., 804-806.

37   Buster, Seed, and Seed et al., *Journal of the American Medical Association*, 1171; Sauer and Buster et al., op. cit.

38   Corea, op. cit., 87.

39 Sauer and Buster et al., op. cit., 805.

40 Ibid.

41 Ibid.

42 Ibid., 806.

43 M. V. Sauer, R. E. Anderson, and R. J. Paulsen, "A trial of superovulation in ovum donors undergoing uterine lavage," *Fertility and Sterility* 51 (January 1989): 131-134.

44 Ibid., 131.

45 Buster and Sauer, op. cit., 46-47.

46 Ramsey, op. cit., 1485.

47 Ibid., 47.

48 Sauer and Buster et al., op. cit., 806.

49 R. G. Edwards, "Chromosomal abnormalities in human embryos," *Nature*, May 26, 1983, 283. See also: R. R. Angell et al., "Chromosome abnormalities in human embryos after in vitro fertilization," *Nature*, May 26, 1983, 336-338; G. Vines, "New insights into early embryos," *New Scientist*, July 9, 1987, 22-23; J. L. Watt et al., "Trisomy 1 in an eight-cell human pre-embryo," *Journal of Medical Genetics* 24 (1987): 60-64; P. M. Summers, J. M. Campbell, and M. W. Miller, "Normal in-vivo development of marmoset monkey embryos after trophectoderm biopsy," *Human Reproduction* 3 (April 1988): 389-393; P. Braude, V. Bolton, and S. Moore, "Human gene expression first occurs between the four- and eight-cell stages of preimplantation development," *Nature*, March 31, 1988, 459-461.

50 R. G. Edwards and D. J. Sharpe, "Social values and research in human embryology," *Nature*, May 14, 1971, 87-88.

51 R. G. Edwards, "Studies in human conception," *American Journal of Obstetrics and Gynecology*, November 1, 1973, 587 and 599.

52 R. G. Edwards and M. Puxon, "Parental consent over embryos," *Nature*, July 19, 1984, 179.

53 K. Johnston, "Sex of new embryos known," *Nature*, June 18, 1987, 547.

54 Ibid.

55 Ibid.

56 A. McLaren, "Can we diagnose genetic disease in pre-embryos?" *New Scientist*, December 10, 1987, 44-45.

57 Ibid., 45.

58 Ibid., 46.

59 Ibid.

60 Ibid.

61 J. Rostand, *Can Man Be Modified?* (New York: Basic Books, 1959), 82-84, 86-87.

FOUR: MAKING THE INSEPARABLE SEPARATE

1 A. Rosenfeld, *The Second Genesis: The Coming Control of Life* (Englewood Cliffs, NJ: Prentice-Hall, 1969), 120.

2 *Life*, "On the frontiers of medicine: control of life," September 10, 1965, 60-61.

3 Ibid., 60.

4 For additional information concerning abortion-related medical experiments, see: A.

Kimbrell, *The Human Body Shop: The Cloning, Engineering, and Marketing of Life* (Washington, DC: Regenery, 1997; D. O'Leary, "Human commodities," *Christianity Today*, March 6, 2000, 58-61.

5   *USA Today*, "Use science to help childless couples," March 9, 1989, 6A.

6   D. P. Alexander, H. G. Britton, and D. A. Nixon, "Maintenance of sheep fetuses by an extracorporeal circuit for periods up to 24 hours," *American Journal of Obstetrics and Gynecology*, December 1, 1968, 969-975.

7   W. M. Zapol et al., "Artificial placenta: two days of total extrauterine support of the isolated premature lamb fetus," *Science*, October 31, 1969, 617-618.

8   Ibid., 618.

9   University of Nebraska Medical Center, *ECMO Parent Information Manual* (Omaha, NE: UNMC, no publication date listed), 5.

10 A. F. Andrews et al., "Venovenous extracorporeal membrane oxygenation (ECMO) using a double-lumen cannula," *Artificial Organs* 11 (June 1987): 265-268; C. R. Redmond et al., "Extracorporeal membrane oxygenation for respiratory and cardiac failure in infants and children," *Journal of Thoracic and Cardiovascular Surgery* 93 (February 1987): 199-204. E. Workman and D. Lentz, "Extracorporeal membrane oxygenation," *AORN Journal* 45 (March 1987): 725-739; R. H. Bartlett et al., "Extracorporeal circulation in neonatal respiratory failure: a prospective randomized study," *Pediatrics* 76 (October 1985): 479-487; N. Paneth and S. Wallenstein, "Extracorporeal membrane oxygenation and the play the winner rule," *Pediatrics* 76 (October 1986): 622-623; D. Arnold et al., "Clinical application of extracorporeal membrane oxygenation (ECMO) in neonatal respiratory failure," *Thoracic and Cardiovascular Surgery* 35 (October 1987): 321-325; R. H. Bartlett et al., "Venovenous perfusion in ECMO for newborn respiratory insufficiency," *Annals in Surgery* 201 (April 1985): 520-526; R. M. Ortiz, R. E. Cilley, and R. H. Bartlett, "Extracorporeal membrane oxygenation in pediatric respiratory failure," *Pediatric Clinics of North America* 34 (February 1987): 39-46.

11 J. M. Toomasian et al., "National experience with extracorporeal membrane oxygenation for newborn respiratory failure," *ASAIO Transcripts* 34 (April-June 1988): 140-147.

12 R. T. Francoeur, "Transformations in Human Reproduction," in Lester A. Kirkendall and Arthur E. Gravatt, eds., *Marriage and Family in the Year 2020* (New York: Prometheus Books, 1984), 95.

13 Ibid.

14 M. Sanger, *Motherhood in Bondage* (New York: Brentano's, 1928), 433.

15 S. Firestone, *The Dialectic of Sex* (New York: William Morrow and Co., 1970), 226.

16 Ibid., 228.

17 Rosenfeld, op. cit., 118.

18 "Doctors aiding women who want to abort on basis of sex," *Lincoln Journal-Star*, December 25, 1988, 9F; B. P. Alter et al., "Prenatal diagnosis of hemoglobinopathies," *New England Journal of Medicine*, December 23, 1976, 1437-1441; "News (gene probes for prenatal diagnosis)," *Birth* 14 (September 1987): 157; D. W. Cox and T. Mansfield, "Prenatal diagnosis of alpha 1 antitrypsin deficiency and estimates of fetal risk for disease," *Journal of Medical Genetics* 24 (1987): 52-59; I. Craft et al., "Multiple pregnancy, selective reduction, and flexible treatment;" *The Lancet*, November 5, 1988, 1087; D. P. Cruikshank et al., "Midtrimester amniocentesis," *American Journal of Obstetrics and Gynecology*, May 15, 1983, 204-211; F. Daffos et al., "Prenatal management of 746 preg-

nancies at risk for toxoplasmosis," *New England Journal of Medicine,* February 4, 1988, 271-275; R. G. Edwards, "Chromosomal abnormalities in human embryos," *Nature,* May 26, 1983, 283; R. G. Edwards and D. J. Sharpe, "Social values and research in human embryology," *Nature,* May 14, 1971, 87-91; J. Elliott, "Abortion for 'wrong' fetal sex: an ethical-legal dilemma," *Journal of the American Medical Association,* October 5, 1979, 1455-1456; M. I. Evans et al., "Selective first trimester termination octuplet and quadruplet pregnancies: clinical and ethical issues," *Obstetrics & Gynecology* 71 (March 1988): 289-296; R. R. Faden et al., "Prenatal screening and pregnant women's attitudes toward the abortion of defective fetuses," *American Journal of Public Health* 77 (November 1987): 288-290; D. F. Farquharson et al., "Management of quintuplet pregnancy by selective embryocide," *American Journal of Obstetrics and Gynecology* 158 (February 1988): 413-416; M. Ferrari et al., "Termination of pregnancy by a dilatation-evacuation technique to obtain placental tissue for DNA analysis," *Prenatal Diagnosis* 8 (March 1988): 235-237; J. C. Fletcher, "Ethics and amniocentesis for sex identification," *The Hastings Center Report,* February 1980, 15-17; R. Frydman et al., "Reduction of the number of embryos in a multiple pregnancy: quintuplet to triplet," *Fertility and Sterility* 48 (1987): 326-327; L. I. Gardner, "Genetically expressed abnormalities in the fetus," *Clinical Obstetrics and Gynecology* 17 (September 1974): 171-193; K. L. Garver, S. L. Marchese, and E. G. Boas, "Amniocentesis," *Obstetrics & Gynecology* 49 (January 1977): 127; F. Gilbert et al., "Prenatal diagnostic options in cystic fibrosis," *American Journal of Obstetrics and Gynecology* 158 (April 1988): 947-952; "Tell us what you think: is it wrong to terminate some fetuses during a multiple pregnancy?" *Glamour,* June 1988, 50; "This is what you thought: 57 percent say a woman should have the right to terminate some fetuses," *Glamour,* September 1988, 197; M. S. Golbus, W. A. Hogge, and S. A. Schonberg, "Chorionic villus sampling: experience of the first 1000 cases," *American Journal of Obstetrics and Gynecology* 154 (June 1986): 1249-1252; M. S. Golbus et al., "Intrauterine diagnosis of genetic defects: results, problems, and follow-up in a prenatal genetic detection center," *American Journal of Obstetrics and Gynecology,* April 1, 1974, 897-905; J. E. Green et al., "Chorionic villus sampling: experience with an initial 940 cases," *Obstetrics & Gynecology* 71 (February 1988): 208-212; L. Grosset, V. Barrelet, and N. Odartchenko, "Antenatal fetal sex determination from maternal blood during early pregnancy," *American Journal of Obstetrics and Gynecology,* September 1, 1974, 60-63; *The Hastings Center Report,* "Prenatal diagnosis for sex choice," February 1980, 20; M. R. Hayden et al., "First-trimester prenatal diagnosis for Huntington's disease with DNA probes," *The Lancet,* June 6, 1987, 1284-1285; R. J. Henry and S. Norton, "Prenatal ultrasound diagnosis of fetal scoliosis with termination of the pregnancy: a case report," *Prenatal Diagnosis* 7 (November 1987): 663-666; W. A. Hogge, "Prenatal diagnosis using DNA probes," *Contemporary OB/GYN,* Technology (1986): 25-31; E. B. Hook and D. M. Scheinemachers, "Trends in utilization of prenatal cytogenetic diagnosis by New York state residents in 1979 and 1980," *American Journal of Public Health* 73 (February 1983): 198-202; C. A. Huether, "Projection of down syndrome births in the United States 1979-2000, and the potential effects of prenatal diagnosis," *American Journal of Public Health* 73 (October 1983): 1186-1189; A. Johnson and L. Goodmilow, "Genetic amniocentesis at 14 weeks or less," *Clinical Obstetrics and Gynecology* 31 (June 1988): 345-352; J. P. Johnson, "Genetic counseling using linked DNA probes: cystic fibrosis as a prototype," *Journal of Pediatrics* 113 (December 1988): 957-963; S. L. Jones, "Decision making in clinical genetics: ethical implications for perinatal nursing practice," *Journal of Perinatal and Neonatal Nursing* 1 (1988): 11-25; H. H. H. Kanhai et al., "Selective termination in quintuplet pregnancy during first trimester," *The Lancet*, June 21, 1986, 1447; *The Lancet*, "Maternal serum-alpha-fetoprotein measurement in antenatal screening for anencephaly and spina bifida in early pregnancy," June 25, 1977, 1323-1332; "Screening for fetal and genetic abnormality," *The Lancet*, December 12, 1987, 1408; "Screening for neural-tube defects," *The Lancet*, June 25, 1977, 1345-1346; N. J. Leschot et al., "Chorionic villi sampling: cytogenetic and clinical findings in 500 pregnancies," *British Medical Journal*, August 15, 1987, 407-410; J. N. Macri et al., "Prenatal diagnosis for neural tube defects," *Journal of the American Medical Association*, September 13, 1976, 1251-1254; M. T. Mennuti and D. M. Main, "Neural tube defects: issues in prenatal diagnosis and counseling," *Obstetrics & Gynecology* 67 (January 1986): 1-16; A. Milunsky et al., "Prenatal diagnosis of neural tube defects," *American Journal of Obstetrics and Gynecology*, April 15, 1982, 1030-1032; P. Miny and W. Holzgreve, "Chorionic villi sampling with an echogenic catheter: experiences of the first 500 cases," *Journal of Perinatal Medicine* 15 (1987): 244-250; P. Miny et al., "Safety of placental biopsy in the second and third trimesters," *New England Journal of Medicine* 317 (No. 18): 1159; B. Modell, "Chorionic villus sampling," *The Lancet*, March 30, 1985, 737-740; H. L. Nader and A. B. Gerbie, "Role of amniocentesis in the intrauterine detection of genetic disorders," *New England Journal of Medicine*, March 12, 1970, 596-599; J. V. Neel, "Some genetic aspects of therapeutic abortion," *Perspectives in Biology and Medicine,* Autumn 1967, 129-135; "Determination of fetal sex early in pregnancy," *New England Journal of Medicine*, October 20, 1983, 979-980; NICHD National Registry for Amniocentesis Study Group, "Midtrimester amniocentesis for prenatal diagnosis," *Journal of the American Medical Association*, September 27, 1976, 1471-1476; C. E. Nugent et al., "Prenatal diagnosis of cystic fibrosis by chorionic villus sampling using 12 polymorphic deoxyribonucleic acid markers," *Obstetrics & Gynecology* 71 (February 1988): 213-215; H. Ostrer and J. Fielding Hejtmancik, "Prenatal diagnosis and carrier detection of genetic diseases by analysis of deoxyribonucleic acid," *Journal of Pediatrics* 112 (May 1988): 679-687; G. E. Palomaki and J. E. Haddow, "Maternal serum alpha-fetoprotein, age, and Down syndrome risk," *American Journal of Obstetrics and Gynecology* 156 (February 1987): 460-463; M. Pembrey, "Embryo transfer in prevention of genetic disease," *The Lancet*, October 13, 1979, 802; B. B. B. K. Pirani et. al., "Amniotic fluid testosterone in the prenatal determination of fetal sex," *American Journal of Obstetrics and Gynecology*, November 1, 1977, 518-520; S. M. Puck and J. P. Fleming, *Genetic Environment and Your Baby: A Workbook for Parents to Be* (Sante Fe, NM: Vivagen, Inc., 1986); O. W. J. Quarrell et al., "Exclusion testing for Huntington's disease in pregnancy with a closely linked DNA marker," *The Lancet*, June 6, 1987, 1281-1283; S. A. Rhine et al., "Prenatal sex detection with endocervical smears: successful results utilizing Y-body fluorescence," *American Journal of Obstetrics and Gynecology*, May 15, 1975, 155-160; B. K. Rothman, *The Tentative Pregnancy: Prenatal Diagnosis and the Future of Motherhood* (New York: Viking/Penguin, 1987); R. H. Schwarz, "Amniocentesis," *Clinical Obstetrics and Gynecology* 18 (June 1975): 1-22; H. F. Selle, D. W. Holmes, and M. L. Ingbar, "The growing demand for midtrimester amniocentesis: a systems approach to forecasting the need for facilities," *American Journal of Public Health* 69 (June 1979): 574-580; M. J. Seller, "Congenital abnormalities and selective abortion," *Journal of Medical Ethics* 2 (1976): 138-141; J. Shaley et al., "Selective reduction of multifetal pregnancies," *New England Journal of Medicine* 319 (1988): 949; B. Siegel, "The promise and problems of prenatal testing," *American Baby*, November 1987, 95-101; J. L. Simpson et al., "Methods for detecting neural tube defects," *Contemporary OB/GYN,* January 1986, 202-222; N. E. Simpson et al., "Prenatal diagnosis of genetic disease in Canada: report of a collaborative study,"

Canadian Medical Association Journal, October 23, 1976, 739-746; D. C. Sokal et al., "Prenatal chromosomal diagnosis: racial and geographic variation in older women in Georgia," *Journal of the American Medical Association,* September 19, 1980, 1355-1357; M. Super et al., "Clinic experience of prenatal diagnosis of cystic fibrosis by use of linked DNA probes," *The Lancet,* October 3, 1987, 782-784; M. S. Verp et al., "Parental decision following prenatal diagnosis of fetal chromosome abnormality," *American Journal of Medical Genetics* 29 (March 1988): 613-622; R. J. Wapner and L. Jackson, "Chorionic villus sampling," *Clinical Obstetrics and Gynecology* 31 (June 1988): 328-344; D. D. Weaver, "A survey of prenatally diagnosed disorders," *Clinical Obstetrics and Gynecology* 31 (June 1988): 253-269; C. P. Weiner," The role of cordocentesis in fetal diagnosis," *Clinical Obstetrics and Gynecology* 31 (June 1988): 285-292; R. H. Williams, "Our role in the generation, modification, and termination of life," *Journal of the American Medical Association,* August 11, 1969, 914-917; R. A. Williamson and J. C. Murray, "Molecular analysis of genetic disorders," *Clinical Obstetrics and Gynecology* 31 (June 1988): 270-284; J. W. Wladimiroff et al., "Prenatal diagnosis of chromosome abnormalities in the presence of fetal structural defects," *American Journal of Medical Genetics* 29 (February 1988): 289-291; S. R. Young et al., "The results of one thousand consecutive prenatal diagnoses," *American Journal of Obstetrics and Gynecology,* September 15, 1983, 181-188.

19   C. S. Lewis, *The Abolition of Man* (New York: Macmillan, 1965), 63.

20   C. S. Lewis, *That Hideous Strength* (New York: Macmillan, 1965), 172-173. Used by permission from William Collins Sons & Co., Ltd., London, England.

FIVE: TO CATCH A FALLING STAR

1   R. J. Lilford and M. E. Dalton, "Effectiveness of treatment for infertility," *British Medical Journal,* July 18, 1987, 155.

2   Committee on Small Business, *Consumer Protection Issues Involving In Vitro Fertilization Clinics* (Washington, DC: U.S. Government Printing Office, 1988), 16.

3   U.S. Congress, Office of Technology Assessment, *Infertility: Medical and Social Choices,* OTA-BA-358. (Washington DC: U.S. Government Printing Office, May 1988), 141.

4   Ibid., 5.

5   D. Harris, "What it costs to fight infertility," *Money,* December 1984, 212.

6   L. J. Lord, "Desperately seeking baby," *U.S. News & World Report,* October 5, 1987, 61.

7   Ibid., 63.

8   R. W. Rebar et al., "Are we exploiting the infertile couple?" *Fertility and Sterility* 48 (November 1987): 735.

9   Harris, op. cit., 202.

10   W. J. Winslade and J. Wilson Ross, *Choosing Life or Death: A Guide for Patients, Families, and Professionals* (New York: The Free Press, 1986), 127-128.

11   B. Kearney, *High-Tech Conception* (New York: Bantam, 1998), 83; Harris, op. cit., 206; U.S. Congress, OTA, op. cit., 141.

12   Medical Economics Co., Inc, *Physician's Desk Reference to Prescription Drugs, 43rd ed., 1989* (Oradell, NJ: Medical Economics, Inc, 1989): 2030-2033; American Hospital Formulary Service, *Drug Information: 1988* (Bethesda, MD: American Society of Hospital Pharmacists, 1988), 2137-2139; United States Pharmacopeial Convention, *USP Dispensing Information, 8th ed., 1988* (Rockville, MD: United States Pharmacopeial

Convention, 1988), 736-737; J. Seligmann, "Do fertility drugs cause cancer?" *Newsweek*, October 10, 1994, 58; M. Lord, "Fear of fertility drugs," *U.S. News & World Report*, May 3, 1993, 81-82; J. Raloff, "Ovarian cancer: homing in on the true risk," *Science News*, July 5, 1997, 7; N. Seppa, "Ovulation cycles linked to ovarian cancer," *Science News*, July 5, 1997, 7; L. K. Altman, "Study uncovers link of cancer to birth drugs," *New York Times* (Late Edition), September 22, 1994, A22; "Fertility drugs may raise ovarian cancer risk," *Journal of the National Cancer Institute*, January 20, 1993 (another report linking fertility drugs to increased ovarian cancer risk was featured in this journal on July 2, 1997); "Ovarian tumors in a cohort of infertile women," *New England Journal of Medicine* 331 (1994): 12; T. Engel et al., "Ovarian hyperstimulation syndrome," *American Journal of Obstetrics and Gynecology*, April 15, 1972, 1052-1060; C. Derom et al., "Increased monozygotic twinning rate after ovulation induction," *The Lancet*, May 30, 1987, 1236-1238; A. MacFarlane et al., "Multiple pregnancy and assisted reproduction," *The Lancet*, November 7, 1987, 1090; J. G. Schenker, S. Yarkoni, and M. Granat, "Multiple pregnancies following induction of ovulation," *Fertility and Sterility* 35 (February 1981): 105-123.

13   United States Pharmacopeial Convention, op. cit, 736; G. E. Schmidt et al., "The effects of enclomiphene and zuclomiphene citrates on mouse embryos fertilized in vitro and in vivo," *American Journal of Obstetrics and Gynecology* 154 (April 1986): 727-736.

14   U. S. Congress, OTA, op. cit., 10.

15   Committee on Small Business, op. cit., 16.

16   U.S. Congress, OTA, op. cit., 131.

17   The Aicardis tell their story in *U.S. News & World Report*, October 5, 1987, 58, 60, 61.

18   U. S. Congress , OTA, op. cit., 4.

19   J. Menken, J. Trussell, and U. Larsen, "Age and infertility," *Science*, September 26, 1986, 1389-1390.

20   U. S. Congress, OTA, op. cit., 3.

21   Menken, Trussell, and Larsen, op. cit., 1391.

22   J. A. Collins et al., "Treatment-independent pregnancy among infertile couples," *New England Journal of Medicine*, November 17, 1983, 1201-1205; See also: D. Berstein et al., "Is conception in infertile couples treatment-related?" *International Journal of Fertility* 24 (1979): 65-67; J. Jarrell et al., "An in vitro fertilization and embryo transfer pilot study: treatment-dependent and treatment-independent pregnancies," *American Journal of Obstetrics and Gynecology* 154 (February 1986): 231-235; S. I. Roh et al., "In vitro fertilization and embryo transfer: treatment-dependent versus -independent pregnancies," *Fertility and Sterility* 48 (December 1987): 982-986.

23   Ibid.

24   Menken, Trussell, and Larsen, op. cit., 1391.

25   R. A. Hatcher et al., *Contraceptive Technology 1988-1989*, 14th rev. ed. (New York: Irvington Publishers, 1988), 37-40, 100-102; A. E. Washington, P. S. Arno, and M. A. Brooks, "The economic cost of pelvic inflammatory disease," *Journal of the American Medical Association*, April 4, 1986, 1735-1738; M. F. Goldsmith, "Sexually transmitted diseases may reverse the 'revolution,'" *Journal of the American Medical Association*, April 4, 1986, 1665-1672; J. Torrington, "Pelvic inflammatory disease," *JOGN Nursing*, Supplement (November/December 1985): 21s-31s; L. Svensson, P. A. Mardh, and L. Westrom, "Infertility after acute salpingitis [PID] with special reference to chlamydia trachomatis," *Fertility and Sterility* 40 (1983): 322-329.

26   Committee on Small Business, op. cit., 16.

27   J. R. Daling et al., "Primal tubal infertility in relation to the use of an intrauterine device," *New England Journal of Medicine*, April 11, 1985, 937-941; D. W. Cramer et al., "Tubal infertility and the intrauterine device," *New England Journal of Medicine*, April 11, 1985, 941-947; W. L. Faulkner and H. W. Ory, "Intrauterine devices and acute pelvic inflammatory disease," *Journal of the American Medical Association*, April 26, 1986, 1851-1853; K. Roberts, "The intrauterine device as a health risk," *Women & Health* 2 (July/August 1977): 21-29; Y. Hata et al., "The effect of long-term use of intrauterine devices," *International Journal of Fertility* 14 (July-September 1969): 241-249; Hatcher et al., op. cit., 101; S. O. Aral, W. D. Mosher, and W. Cates, Jr., "Contraceptive use, pelvic inflammatory disease, and fertility problems among American women," *American Journal of Obstetrics and Gynecology* 256 (1987): 59-64; N. C. Lee, G. L. Rubin, and H. W. Ory, "Type of intrauterine device and the risk of pelvic inflammatory disease," *Obstetrics & Gynecology* 62 (1983): 1-6.

28   L. J. Lord, op. cit., 59.

29   Hatcher et al., op. cit., 101.

30   A. E. Washington et al., "Oral contraceptives, chlamydia trachomatis infection, and pelvic inflammatory disease: a word of caution about protection," *Journal of the American Medical Association*, April 19, 1985, 2246-2250; D. W. Cramer et al., "The relationship of tubal infertility to barrier method and oral contraceptive use," *Journal of the American Medical Association*, May 8, 1987, 2446-2450.

31   C. J. Hogue, W. Cates, and C. Tietze, "Effects of induced abortion on subsequent reproduction," *Epidemiological Review* 4 (1982): 66-94.

32   W. R. Phipps, D. W. Cramer, and I. Schiff, "The association between smoking and female infertility as influenced by the cause of the infertility," *Fertility and Sterility* 48 (1987): 377-382; R. J. Stillman, M. J. Rosenberg, and B. P. Sachs, "Smoking and reproduction," *Fertility and Sterility* 46 (1986): 545; A. J. Hartz et al., "The association of smoking with clinical indicators of altered sex steroids—a study of 50,145 women," *Public Health Reports* 102 (1987): 254-259; A. Wilcox, C. Weinberg, and D. Baird, "Caffeinated beverages and decreased fertility," *The Lancet*, December 24/31, 1988, 1453-1456.

33   J. Wyngaarden, "Study finds association between smoking and certain types of infertility," *Journal of the American Medical Association*, July 8, 1988, 161.

34   D. D. Baird and A. J. Wilcox, "Cigarette smoking with delayed conception," *Journal of the American Medical Association*, May 24/31, 1985, 2979-2983.

35   Wilcox, Weinberg, and Baird, op. cit, 1453.

36   U. S. Congress, OTA, op. cit., 63-64; B. A. Bullen et al., "Induction of menstrual disorders by strenuous exercise in untrained women," *New England Journal of Medicine*, 1985, 1345-1353; P. T. Ellison and C. Lager, "Moderate recreational running is associated with lowered salivary progesterone profiles in women," *American Journal of Obstetrics and Gynecology* 154 (1986): 1000-1003; Z. M. Van Der Spuy, "Nutrition and reproduction," *Clinics in Obstetrics and Gynecology* 12 (1985): 579-604; R. E. Frisch, "Body fat, puberty, and fertility," *Science* 185 (1984): 949-953; M. Seibel and M. Taynor, "Emotional aspects of infertility," *Fertility and Sterility* 37 (1982): 137-145.

37   Committee on Small Business, op. cit., 16.

38   G. Sher, V. M. Davis, J. Stoess, *In Vitro Fertilization: The ART of Making Babies* (New York: Facts on File, 1998), xiv, xvi, 185.

39   P. Neumann, S. Gharib, and M. Weinstein, "The cost of a successful delivery with in vitro fertilization," *New England Journal of Medicine* 331 (1994): 240.

40   Menken, Trussell, and Larsen, op. cit., 1393.

41   M. Potts and D. A. Grimes, "STDs, IVF, and barrier contraception (Letter)," *Journal of the American Medical Association*, October 2, 1987, 1729.

42   L. J. Lord, op. cit., 58.

43   U.S. Congress, OTA, op. cit., 141.

44   *Wisconsin Medical Journal* 87 (March 1988): 63.

45   S. O. Aral and W. Cates, "The increasing concern with infertility: why now?" *Journal of the American Medical Association*, November 4, 1983, 2330.

46   Information obtained by phone from the American College of Obstetricians and Gynecologists.

47   Aral and Cates, op. cit., 2330.

48   L. J. Lord, op. cit., 59.

SIX: WHEN TO SAY STOP

1   C . S. Lewis, *The Abolition of Man* (New York: Macmillan, 1955), 71.

2   Roger Gosden, *Designing Babies* (New York: W. H. Freeman, 1999), 5.

3   Portions of this chapter and Appendix B are adapted from articles I have written for publication in *Christian Parenting Today* and *Clarity* magazines and two books I have authored: *Blessed Events: Christian Couples Share Their Experiences of God's Blessing Through Infertility, Natural Parenting, and Adoption* (Wheaton, IL: Crossway, 1990) and *The Christian Woman's Guide to Personal Health Care* (Wheaton, IL: Crossway, 1998). Unless otherwise noted, quotes in this chapter are from phone conversations during my research.

4   Debra Evans, *Blessed Events: Christian Couples Share Their Experiences of God's Blessing Through Infertility, Natural Parenting, and Adoption* (Wheaton, IL: Crossway, 1990), 85-93.

5   A. Baran and R. Pannor, *Lethal Secrets: The Shocking Consequences and Unsolved Problems of Artificial Insemination* (New York: Warner, 1989), 25.

6   Sue Halpern, "Infertility: playing the odds," *Ms.*, January/February 1989, 148.

7   Committee on Government Operations, *Medical and Social Choices for Infertile Couples and the Federal Role in Prevention and Treatment* (Washington, DC: U.S. Government Printing Office, 1989), 48-49.

8   Halpern, op cit.

9   U.S. Congress, Office of Technology Assessment, *Infertility: Medical and Social Choices* (Washington DC: U.S. Government Printing Office, May 1988, OTA-BA-358); W. D. Mosher and W. F. Pratt, "Fecundity and infertility in the United States, 1965-1988," advance data from *Vital Health Statistics of the National Center for Health Statistics*, December 4, 1990, 1.

10   G. Cowley, "Made to order babies," *Newsweek*, Winter/Spring 1990, 98.

11   For a review of the history of IVF research, see: J. Rock and A. T. Hertig: "Some aspects of early human development," *American Journal of Obstetrics and Gynecology* 44 (1942):973-983; J. Rock and M. F. Menkin, "In vitro fertilization and cleavage of human ovarian eggs," *Science*, August 4, 1944, 105; M. F. Menkin and J. Rock: "In vitro fertil-

ization and cleavage of human ovarian eggs," *American Journal of Obstetrics and Gynecology* 55 (1948): 440-454; A. T. Hertig, "A fifteen-year search for first-stage human ova," *Journal of the American Medical Association*, January 20, 1989, 434-435; R. G. Edwards, "Maturation in vitro of mouse, sheep, cow, pig, rhesus monkey and human ovarian oocytes," *Nature*, October 23, 1965, 349-351; R. G. Edwards, "Maturation in vitro of human ovarian oocytes," *The Lancet*, November 6, 1965, 926-929; R. G. Edwards, B. D. Bavister, and P. C. Steptoe, "Early stages of fertilization in vitro of human oocytes matured in vitro," *Nature*, February 15, 1969, 632-635; R. G. Edwards, "Mammalian eggs in the laboratory," *Scientific American* 215 (1966): 81; R. G. Edwards, B. D. Bavister, and P. C. Steptoe, "Early stages of fertilization *in vitro* of human oocytes matured *in vitro*," *Nature*, February 15, 1969, 632; L. Shettles, "Observations on human follicular and tubal ova," *American Journal of Obstetrics and Gynecology*, 1953, 66(2): 235-247; L. Shettles, "A morula stage of human ova developed in vitro," *Fertility and Sterility*, 1955, 6(4): 287-289; L. Shettles: "Corona radiata and zona pellucida of living human ova," *Fertility and Sterility*, 1958, 9(2): 167-170; L. Mastroianni and C. Noriega, "Observations on human ova and the fertilization process," *American Journal of Obstetrics and Gynecology*, 1970, 107(5): 682-690; J. F. Kennedy and R. P. Donahue, "Human oocytes: maturation in chemically defined media," *Science* 164 (June 13, 1969): 1292-1293; P. Liedholm, P. Sundstrom, and H. Wramsky, "A model for experimental studies on human egg transfer," *Archives of Andrology*, 1980, 5(1): 92; L. McLaughlin, *The Pill, John Rock and the Church* (Boston: Little, Brown and Company, 1982); R. G. Edwards and P. Steptoe, *A Matter of Life* (New York: William Morrow, 1980); R. G. Edwards and R. E. Fowler, "Human embryos in the laboratory," *Scientific American* 223 (1970): 50; R. G. Seed, R. W. Seed, and D. S. Baker, "Aspects of bovine embryo transplant directly applicable to humans: a report of over 300 procedures," *Fertility and Sterility* 28 (March 1977): 313-314; R. G. Seed and R. W. Seed, "Artificial embryonation: human embryo transplant," *Archives in Andrology* 5 (1980): 90-91.

For studies involving embryo research, see: J. E. Buster, R. W. Seed, and R. G. Seed et al., "Nonsurgical ovum transfer as a treatment in infertile women," *Journal of the American Medical Association*, March 2, 1984, 1171-1173; J. E. Buster et al., "An instrument for the recovery of preimplantation uterine ova," *Obstetrics & Gynecology* 71 (May 1988): 804-806; J. E. Buster, R. W. Seed, and R. G. Seed et al., "Nonsurgical ovum transfer of in vivo fertilized donated ova to five infertile women: report of two pregnancies," *The Lancet*, July 23, 1983, 223-224; M. V. Sauer, R. E. Anderson, and R. J. Paulsen, "A trial of superovulation in ovum donors undergoing uterine lavage," *Fertility and Sterility* 51 (January 1989): 131-134; J. D. Biggers, "In vitro fertilization and embryo transfer in human beings," *New England Journal of Medicine,* February 5, 1981, 336-341; A. Trounson and L. Mohr, "Human pregnancy following cryopreservation, thawing and transfer of an eight-cell embryo," *Nature*, October 20, 1983, 707-709; A. Trounson, "Pregnancy established in an infertile patient after transfer of a donated embryo fertilized in vitro," *British Medical Journal*, March 12, 1983, 835-838; A. Trounson et al., "Effect of growth in culture medium on the rate of mouse embryo development and viability in vitro," *Journal of In Vitro Fertilization and Embryo Transfer* 4 (October 1987): 265-268; A. Trounson, "Preservation of human eggs and embryos," *Fertility and Sterility* 46 (July 1986): 1-11; A. Trounson, A. Peura, and C. Kirby, "Ultrarapid freezing: a new low-cost and effective method of embryo cryopreservation," *Fertility and Sterility* 48 (November 1987): 843-850; A. Trounson et al., "Ultrarapid freezing of early cleavage stage human embryos and eight-cell mouse embryos," *Fertility and Sterility* 49 (May 1988): 822-826; S. A. Hassani et al., "Cryopreservation of human oocytes," *Human*

Reproduction 2 (November 1987): 695-700; A. Clark et al., "Social and reproductive characteristics of the first 100 couples treated by in-vitro fertilization programme at National Women's Hospital, Auckland," *New Zealand Medical Journal*, June 24, 1987, 380-382; "Success rates for IVF and GIFT," *Contemporary OB/GYN*, May 1988, 89-106; J. E. Buster and M. V. Sauer, "Nonsurgical donor ovum transfer: new option for infertile couples," *Contemporary OB/GYN*, August 1986, 39-49; I. Craft et al., "Analysis of 1071 GIFT procedures: the case for a flexible approach to treatment," *The Lancet*, May 16, 1988, 1094-1097; I. Craft et al., "Successful pregnancies from the transfer of pronucleate embryos in an outpatient in vitro fertilization program," *Fertility and Sterility* 44 (August 1985): 181-184; A. H. DeCherney and G. Lavy, "Oocyte recovery methods in in-vitro fertilization," *Clinical Obstetrics and Gynecology* 29 (March 1986): 171-179; J. Deschacht et al., "In vitro fertilization with husband and donor sperm in patients with previous fertilization failures using husband sperm," *Human Reproduction* 3 (January 1988): 105-108; R. Frydman et al., "A new approach to follicular stimulation for in vitro fertilization: programmed oocyte retrieval," *Fertility and Sterility* 46 (October 1986): 657-659; R. Frydman et al., "An obstetric assessment of the first 100 births from the in vitro fertilization program at Clamart, France," *American Journal of Obstetrics and Gynecology* 154 (March 1986): 550-555; R. Frydman et al., "Programmed oocyte retrieval during routine laparoscopy and embryo cryopreservation for later transfer," *American Journal of Obstetrics and Gynecology* 155 (July 1986): 112-117; H. Jones et al., "An analysis of the obstetric outcome of 125 consecutive pregnancies conceived in vitro and resulting in 100 deliveries," *American Journal of Obstetrics and Gynecology* 154 (April 1986): 848-854; H. Jones, H. Liu, and Z. Rosenwaks, "The efficiency of human reproduction after in vitro fertilization and embryo transfer," *Fertility and Sterility* 49 (1988): 649-653; H. Jones et al., "The program for in vitro fertilization at Norfolk," *Fertility and Sterility* 38 (1982):14-20; J. Leeton, A. Trounson, D. Jessup, and C. Wood, "The technique for embryo transfer," *Fertility and Sterility* 38 (1982):156-161; "100 test-tube babies gather in Baltimore," *Lincoln Journal*, September 12, 1988, 6; "In vitro clinics span globe; spawn new treatments," *Lincoln Sunday Journal-Star*, July 24, 1988, 1A, 6A; R. P. Marrs, "Human in-vitro fertilization," *Clinical Obstetrics and Gynecology* 29 (March 1986): 117; R. P. Marrs, "Laboratory conditions for human in-vitro fertilization procedures," *Clinical Obstetrics and Gynecology* 29 (March 1986): 180-189; Medical Research International and the American Fertility Society Special Interest Group, "In vitro fertilization/embryo transfer in the united states: 1985 and 1986, results from the national IVF/ET registry," *Fertility and Sterility* 49 (February 1988): 212-215; D. R. Meldrum et al., "Evolution of a highly successful in vitro fertilization-embryo transfer program," *Fertility and Sterility* 48 (July 1987): 86-93; S. Pace-Owens, "In vitro fertilization and embryo transfer," *JOGN Nursing*, Supplement (November/December 1985): 44S-48S; C. Ranoux et al., "A new in vitro fertilization technique: intravaginal culture," *Fertility and Sterility* 49 (April 1988): 654-657; C. Ranoux et al., "Intravaginal culture and embryo transfer: a new method for the fertilization of human oocytes," *Review of French Gynecology and Obstetrics* 82 (December 1987): 741-744; J. M. Rary et. al., "Techniques of in vitro fertilization of oocytes and embryo transfer in humans," *Archives of Andrology* 5 (1980): 89-90; V. Sharma et al., "An analysis of factors influencing the establishment of a clinical pregnancy in an ultrasound-based ambulatory in vitro fertilization clinic," *Fertility and Sterility* 49 (March 1988): 468-478; P. H. Wessels et al., "Gamete intrafallopian transfer: a treatment for long-standing infertility," *Journal of In Vitro Fertilization and Embryo Transfer* 4 (October 1987): 256-259; C. Wood et al., "Clinical features of eight pregnancies resulting from in vitro fertilization and embryo transfer," *Fertility and Sterility* 38 (July 1982): 22; C. Wood et al., "Factors influencing pregnancy rates following in vitro fertilization and embryo transfer," *Fertility and Sterility* 43 (1985): 245-250.

12 R. G. Edwards, "The case for studying human embryos and their constituent tissues in vitro," in *Human Conception In Vitro*, R. G. Edwards and J. Purdy, eds. (London: Academic Press, date unknown), 372.

13 K. Dawson, "Introduction," in *Embryo Experimentation: Ethical, Legal, and Social Issues*, P. Singer, H. Kuhse, S. Buckle, K. Dawson, and P. Kasimba, eds. (New York: Cambridge University Press, 1990), xv.

14 T. Iglesias, *A Basic Ethic for Man's Well-Being: Conscience and the New Scientific Possibilities* (Southport, Merseyside, GB: Gowland & Co., 1989), 12.

15 Ibid.

16 Ibid., 24.

17 G. Kolata, "In vitro fertilization goes commercial," *Science* 221 (1983): 1160-1161; F. S. Chapman, "Going for the gold in the baby business," *Fortune*, September 17, 1984, 41; M. Novak, "Buying & selling babies: limitations on the marketplace," *Commonweal*, July 17, 1987, 406-407; G. Annas, "Making babies without sex: the law and the profits," *American Journal of Public Health* 74 (December 1984): 1415-1417; "Babies: No Sale," *Los Angeles Times*, February 4, 1988; C. A. Raymond, "IVF registry notes more centers, more births, slightly improved odds," *Journal of the American Medical Association*, April 1, 1988, 1920-1921; Committee on Small Business, *Consumer Protection Issues Involving In Vitro Fertilization Clinics* (Washington, DC: U.S. Government Printing Office, 1988); A. Taylor Fleming, "New frontiers in conception," *New York Times Magazine*, July 20, 1980; G. Annas, "Redefining parenthood and protecting embryos: why we need new laws," *The Hastings Center Report*, October 1984, 50-52; G. Annas and S. Elias, "Social policy considerations in noncoital reproduction," *Journal of the American Medical Association*, January 3, 1986, 62-68; P. Bagne, "High-tech breeding," *Mother Jones* 8 (August 1983): 23-29, 35; H. Jones, Jr., "The impact of in vitro fertilization on the practice of gynecology and obstetrics," *International Journal of Fertility* 31 (1986): 99-111; J. E. Buster and M. V. Sauer, "Nonsurgical donor ovum transfer: New option for infertile couples," *Contemporary OB/GYN*, August 1986, 39-49; "Ovum donor transfer may see wide use in treating infertility," *Ob/Gyn News*, December 1, 1983, 1.

18 A. Kimbrell, *The Human Body Shop: The Cloning, Engineering, and Marketing of Life* (Washington, DC: Regnery, 1997), 79.

19 A. L. Cowan, "Can a baby-making venture deliver?" *New York Times*, June 1, 1992, D1, D6.

20 Ibid.

21 P. J. Nuemann, S. D. Gharb, and M. C. Weinstein, "The cost of a successful delivery with in vitro fertilization," *New England Journal of Medicine* 331 (1994): 239-243.

22 J. Robertson, *Children of Choice* (Princeton, NJ: Princeton University Press, 1994), 99.

23 L. Andrews, *The Clone Age: Adventures in the New World of Reproductive Technology* (New York: Henry Holt, 1999), 35.

24 P. Ramsey, "Shall we 'reproduce'? Part I. The medical ethics of in vitro fertilization," *Journal of the American Medical Association*, June 5, 1972, 1346-1350; P. Ramsey, "Shall we 'reproduce'? Part II. Rejoinders and future forecast," *Journal of the American Medical Association*, June 12, 1972, 1484-1485; P. Ramsey, *Fabricated Man* (New Haven, CT:

Yale University Press, 1970); R. G. Edwards, "Chromosomal abnormalities in human embryos," *Nature*, May 26, 1983, 283; R. R. Angell et al., "Chromosome abnormalities in human embryos after in vitro fertilization," *Nature*, May 26, 1983, 336-338; G. Vines, "New insights into early embryos," *New Scientist*, July 9, 1987, 22-23; J. L. Watt et al., "Trisomy 1 in an eight-cell human pre-embryo," *Journal of Medical Genetics* 24 (1987): 60-64; P. M. Summers, J. M. Campbell, and M. W. Miller, "Normal in-vivo development of marmoset monkey embryos after trophectoderm biopsy," *Human Reproduction* 3 (April 1988): 389-393; P. Braude, V. Bolton, and S. Moore, "Human gene expression first occurs between the four- and eight-cell stages of preimplantation development," *Nature*, March 31, 1988, 459-461; R. G. Edwards and D. J. Sharpe, "Social values and research in human embryology," *Nature*, May 14, 1971, 87-88; R. G. Edwards, "Studies in human conception," *American Journal of Obstetrics and Gynecology*, November 1, 1973, 587, 599; R. G. Edwards and M. Puxon, "Parental consent over embryos," *Nature*, July 19, 1984, 179; K. Johnston, "Sex of new embryos known," *Nature*, June 18, 1987, 547; A. McLaren, "Can we diagnose genetic disease in pre-embryos?" *New Scientist*, December 10, 1987, 44-45.

25   Kimbrell, *Human Body Shop*, 143-144.

26   Ibid., 144.

27   J. Ashkenazi et al., "Abdominal complications following ultrasonically guided percutaneous transvesical collection of oocytes for in vitro fertilization," *Journal of In Vitro Fertilization and Embryo Transfer* 4 (December 1987): 316-318; J. Ashkenasi et al., "Multiple pregnancy after in-vitro fertilization and embryo transfer: report of a quadruplet pregnancy and delivery," *Human Reproduction* 2 (August 1987): 511-515; F. R. Batzer et al., "Multiple pregnancies with gamete intrafallopian transfer (gift): complications of a new technique," *Journal of In Vitro Fertilization and Embryo Transfer* 5 (February 1988): 35-37; G. Byrne, "Artificial insemination report prompts call for regulation," *Science*, August 19, 1988, 895; E. Chargaff, "Engineering a molecular nightmare," *Nature*, May 21, 1987, 199-200; H. Bequaert Holmes, "In vitro fertilization: reflections on the state of the art," *Birth* 15 (1988): 1134-1144; W. R. Phipps, C. B. Benson, and P. M. McShane, "Severe thigh myositis following intramuscular progesterone injections in an in vitro fertilization patient," *Fertility and Sterility* 49 (March 1988): 536-537; F. V. Price, "The risk of high multiparity with IVF/ET," *Birth* 15 (September 1988): 157-163; J. J. Schlesselman, "How does one assess the risk of abnormalities from human in vitro fertilization?" *American Journal of Obstetrics and Gynecology*, September 1, 1979, 135-148; D. H. Smith et al., "Tubal pregnancy occurring after successful in vitro fertilization and embryo transfer," *Fertility and Sterility* 38 (July 1982): 105-106; J. L. Yovich, S. R. Turner, and A. J. Murphy, "Embryo transfer technique as a cause of ectopic pregnancies in in vitro fertilization," *Fertility and Sterility* 44 (September 1985): 318-321.

28   As quoted in the *Atlanta-Journal Constitution*, October 27, 1991.

29   T. L. Callahan et al., "The economic impact of multiple-gestation pregnancies and the contribution of assisted-reproduction techniques to their incidence," *New England Journal of Medicine* 331 (1994): 244-249; N. Bollen et al., "The incidence of multiple pregnancy after in vitro fertilization and embryo transfer, gamete, or zygote intrafallopian transfer," *Fertility and Sterility* 55 (1991): 314-318; Andrews, *The Clone Age*, 52; M. S. Rein, R. L. Barbieri, and M. F. Greene, "The causes of high-order multiple gestation," *International Journal of Fertility* 35 (1990): 154-156.

30   B. J. Botting, I. M. Davies, and A. J. Macfarlane, "Recent trends in the incidence of mul-

tiple births and associated mortality," *Archives of Diseases in Childhood* 62 (1987): 941-950; Grutzner-Konnecke et al., "Higher order multiple births: natural wonder or failure of therapy?" *ACTA Genetics (Roma)* 39 (1990): 491-495; Andrews, *The Clone Age*, 52-55; J. L. Kiely, J. C. Kleinman, and M. Kiely, "Triplets and higher-order multiple births: time trends and infant mortality," *American Journal of Diseases in Childhood* 146 (1992): 862-868.

31 H. H. H. Kanhai et al., "Selective termination in quintuplet pregnancy during first trimester," *The Lancet*, June 21, 1986, 1447; D. F. Farquharson et al., "Management of quintuplet pregnancy by selective embryocide," *American Journal of Obstetrics and Gynecology* 158 (February 1988): 413-416; M. I. Evans et al., "Selective first trimester termination octuplet and quadruplet pregnancies: clinical and ethical issues," *Obstetrics & Gynecology* 71 (March 1988): 289-296; R. L. Berkowitz et al., "Selective reduction of multifetal pregnancies in the first trimester," *New England Journal of Medicine*, April 21, 1988, 1043-1047; R. L. Berkowitz et al., "Selective reduction of multifetal pregnancies (Reply)," *New England Journal of Medicine*, October 6, 1988, 950-951; J. M. Lorenz and J. S. Terry, "Selective reduction of multifetal pregnancies (Letter)," *New England Journal of Medicine*, October 6, 1988, 949-950; S. L. Romney, "Selective reduction of multifetal pregnancies (Letter)," *New England Journal of Medicine*, October 6, 1988, 949; J. Shalev et al., "Selective reduction of multifetal pregnancies (Letter)," *New England Journal of Medicine*, October 6, 1988, 949; E. F. Diamond, "Selective reduction of multifetal pregnancies (Letter)," *New England Journal of Medicine*, October 6, 1988, 950; D. H. James, "Selective reduction of multifetal pregnancies (Letter)," *New England Journal of Medicine*, October 6, 1988, 950; I. Craft et al., "Multiple pregnancy, selective reduction, and flexible treatment," *The Lancet*, November 5, 1988, 1087; "Selective fetus destruction debated," *Lincoln Journal*, April 21, 1988, A5.

To find out how this subject is being detoxified for presentation in popular women's magazines, see: "Tell us what you think: is it wrong to terminate some fetuses during a multiple pregnancy?" *Glamour*, July 1988, 50; "This is what you thought: 57 percent say a woman should have the right to terminate some fetuses," *Glamour*, September 1988, 197; "Choices," *Woman's World*, January 3, 1989, 44-45; R. Frydman et al., "Reduction of the number of embryos in a multiple pregnancy: from quintuplet to triplet," *Fertility and Sterility* 48 (August 1987): 326-327.

32 Quoted in B. Kearney, *High-Tech Conception* (New York: Bantam, 1998), 281.

33 G. Sher, V. M. Davis, and J. Stoess, *In Vitro Fertilization: The A.R.T. of Making Babies* (New York: Facts on File, 1998), 45, 47.

34 Andrews, *The Clone Age*, 57.

35 L. Silver, *Remaking Eden: How Genetic Engineering and Cloning Will Transform the American Family* (New York: Avon, 1997), 79.

36 K. Dawson, "Introduction: An outline of scientific aspects of embryo research," in *Embryo Experimentation*, op. cit., 3-16.

37 Gene therapy does not affect genetic inheritance, but provides a functional gene as a replacement for a nonfunctional gene. Germ-line engineering, however, fundamentally alters the genetic constitution of a specific person/embryo, thus provoking a permanent change in a person's genetic makeup that will be passed on to future offspring. Numerous scientists have voiced their concerns about germ-line engineering due to its ability to transform individuals over successive generations into a new species, a so-called super-race that could no longer mate successfully with members of the original

(*Homo sapiens*) group. (See L. Silver, *Remaking Eden,* and F. Dyson, *The Sun, the Genome, and the Internet.*)

38   Dawson, "Introduction," *Embryo Experimentation,* 3.

39   Quoted by C. Colson, "Genocide of the Unborn: The Problem with Stem Cell Research," *BreakPoint Commentary,* #000207 - 02/07/2000.

40   R. G. Seed and R. Weiss, "Embryo adoption: technical, ethical and legal aspects," *Archives in Andrology* 5 (1980); D. J. Cuisine, "Some legal implications of embryo transfer," *The Lancet,* August 25, 1979, 407-408; J. E. Buster et al., "Survey of attitudes regarding the use of siblings for gamete donation," *Fertility and Sterility* 49 (April 1988): 721-722; H. I. Abdalla and T. Leonard, "Cryopreserved zygote intrafallopian transfer for anonymous oocyte donation," *The Lancet,* April 9, 1988, 835; American Fertility Society Committee on Ethics, "Donor eggs in in vitro fertilization," *Fertility and Sterility* 46 (September 1986), Supplement 1: 42S-44S; American Fertility Society Committee on Ethics, "Donor sperm in in vitro fertilization," *Fertility and Sterility* 46 (September 1986), Supplement 1: 39S-41S; American Fertility Society Committee on Ethics, "Surrogate gestational mothers: women who gestate a genetically unrelated embryo," *Fertility and Sterility* 46 (September 1986), Supplement 1: 58S-61S; L. B. Andrews, "Embryo technology," *Parent's Magazine* 56 (May 1981): 63-71; L. B. Andrews, "Legal and ethical aspects of new reproductive technologies," *Clinical Obstetrics and Gynecology* 29 (March 1986): 190-204; G. Annas and J. F. Henahan, "Fertilization, embryo transfer procedures raise many questions," *Journal of the American Medical Association,* August 17, 1984, 877-879, 882; J. E. Buster, "Survey of attitudes regarding the use of siblings for gamete donation," *Fertility and Sterility* 49 (April 1988): 721-722; J. F. Correy, "Donor oocyte pregnancy with transfer of deep-frozen embryo," *Fertility and Sterility* 49 (March 1988): 534-535; I. Craft and J. Yovich, "Implications of embryo transfer," *The Lancet,* September 22, 1979, 642-643; I. Craft and P. F. Serhal, "Ovum donation—a simplified approach," *Fertility and Sterility* 48 (August 1987): 265-269; D. J. Cuisine, "Some legal implications of embryo transfer," *The Lancet,* August 25, 1979, 407-408; "What are the moral rights of frozen embryos?" *Health Progress,* October 1984, 54, 62; M. Johnston, "I gave birth to another woman's baby," *Redbook,* May 1984, 44 and 46; A. M. Junca et al., "Anonymous and non-anonymous oocyte donation preliminary results," *Human Reproduction* 3 (January 1988): 121-123; J. F. Leeton et al., "Donor oocyte pregnancy with transfer of deep-frozen embryo," *Fertility and Sterility* 49 (March 1988): 534-535; J. F. Leeton et al., "Successful pregnancy in an ovulating recipient following the transfer of two frozen-thawed embryos obtained from anonymously donated oocytes," *Journal of In Vitro Fertilization and Embryo Transfer* 5 (February 1988): 22-24; J. Leeton and J. Harman, "The donation of oocytes to known recipients," *Australia and New Zealand Journal of Obstetrics and Gynaecology* 27 (August 1987): 248-250; "Woman bears own grandchild," *Lincoln Journal,* October 1, 1987, 2; M. Madhevan, A. O. Trounson, and J. F. Leeton, "Successful use of human semen cryobanking for in vitro fertilization," *Fertility and Sterility* 40 (September 1983): 340-343; M. C. Michelow, "Mother-daughter in vitro fertilization triplet surrogate pregnancy," *Journal of In Vitro Fertilization and Embryo Transfer* 5 (February 1988): 31-34; J. Salat-Baroux et al., "Pregnancies after replacement of frozen-thawed embryos in a donation program," *Fertility and Sterility* 49 (March 1988): 817-821; R. G. Seed and R. W. Seed, "Embryo adoption—technical, ethical and legal aspects," *Archives in Andrology* 5 (1980).

41   J. T. Noonan, "Christian Tradition and the Control of Reproduction," in *The Death Decision,* ed. L. J. Nelson (Ann Arbor, MI: Servant Books, 1984), 14.

42 U.S. Congress, Office of Technology Assessment, *Artificial Insemination Practice in the United States, Summary of a 1987 Survey-Background Paper, OTA-BP-BA-48* (Washington, DC: U.S. Government Printing Office, August 1988), 3, 4, 15, 16.

43 L. B. Andrews, "Yours, mine and theirs," *Psychology Today*, December 1984.

44 S. Robinson and H. F. Pizer, *Having a Baby Without a Man* (New York: Simon & Schuster/ Fireside Books, 1987).

45 Kimbrell, op cit., 87.

46 Andrews, *The Clone Age*, 81.

47 R. Herman, "When the 'father' is a sperm donor," *Washington Post*, February 11, 1992, 13.

48 Andrews, *The Clone Age*, 81.

49 OTA, *Infertility: Medical and Social Choices*, 229.

50 OTA, *Artificial Insemination*, 40.

51 Ibid., 67.

52 Ibid., 41.

53 S. Robinson and H. F. Pizer, op cit.; G. Hanscombe, "The right to lesbian parenthood," *Journal of Medical Ethics* 9 (1983): 133-135; B. Kritchevsky, "The unmarried woman's right to artificial insemination: a call for expanded definition of family," *Harvard Women's Law Journal* 4 (1981): 1-42; Lambda Legal Defense and Education Fund, Inc., Lesbian Rights Project (San Francisco), Office of Gay and Lesbian Health Concerns (NYC Department of Health), and New York University Women's Center, *Lesbians Choosing Motherhood* (New York: Lambda Legal Defense and Education Fund, Inc., 1984); Lesbian Health Information Project, *Artificial Insemination: An Alternative Conception for the Lesbian and Gay Community* (San Francisco, CA: San Francisco Women's Centers, 1979); S. Stern, "Lesbian insemination," *The CoEvolution Quarterly*, Summer 1980, 108-117.

54 Kimbrell, *Human Body Shop*, 88.

55 R. Sharpe, "Love can't take away pain of sperm donor's offspring," *El Paso Times*, December 21, 1986, 24A.

56 OTA, *Artificial Insemination*, 32, 33.

57 Andrews, *The Clone Age*, 80-81.

58 Herman, op cit., 12.

59 R. Fitzhugh, "Where's poppa?" *US Magazine*, October 22, 1984, 68-69. For a detailed discussion on the implications of deception about one's origins, read: A Baran and R. Pannor, *Lethal Secrets: The Shocking Consequences and Unsolved Problems of Artificial Insemination* (New York: Warner, 1989).

60 S. Callahan, "Lovemaking and babymaking," *Commonweal*, April 24, 1987, 237; S. Callahan, "Use of third-party donors threatens basic values," *Health Progress*, March 1987, 26-28; C. Krauthammer, "The ethics of human manufacture," *The New Republic*, May 4, 1987, 17-21; B. Katz Rothman, "How science is redefining parenthood," *Ms.*, July/August 1982, 154, 156; A. Baran and R. Pannor, *Lethal Secrets: The Shocking Consequences and Unsolved Problem of Artificial Insemination* (New York: Warner, 1989); H. J. Muller, "Human evolution by voluntary choice of germ plasm," *Science*, September 8, 1961, 643-649; H. D. Krause, "Artificial conception, legislative approaches," *Family Law Quarterly* 19 (Fall 1988): 185-206; R. P. S. Jansen, "Sperm and ova as property," *Journal of Medical Ethics* 11 (1985): 123-126; R. Snowden and G. D. Mitchell, *Artificial Reproduction: A Social Investigation* (London: George Allen & Unwin, 1983); L. B. Andrews, *New Conceptions*

(New York: Ballantine Books, 1985); R. Snowden and G. D. Mitchell, *The Artificial Family: A Consideration of Artificial Insemination by Donor* (London: George Allen & Unwin, 1981); R. C. Strickler, D. W. Keller, and J. C. Warren, "Artificial insemination with fresh donor semen," *New England Journal of Medicine,* October 23, 1975, 848-853; J. L. Yovich, "Surrogacy," *The Lancet,* June 13, 1987, 1374; M. Curie-Cohen, L. Luttrell, and S. Shapiro, "Current practice of artificial insemination by donor in the United States," *New England Journal of Medicine,* March 15, 1979, 585-590.

SEVEN: PRESENT AND FUTURE POSSIBILITIES

1   Quoted in L. Kass, *Toward a More Natural Science* (New York: The Free Press, 1985), 318.

2   "Reflections," *Christianity Today,* March 17, 1989, 33.

3   "UK agonizes over embryo research," *Nature,* February 7, 1985, 424; "Warnock proposals in trouble," *Nature,* February 7, 1985, 417; H. J. Evans and A. McLaren, "Unborn children (protection) bill," *Nature,* March 14, 1985, 127-128; "Britain hazards embryo research," *Nature,* December 3, 1987, 407; S. Hadlington, "British government hedges bets on embryo research," *Nature,* December 3, 1987, 409; "Research on human embryos," *The Lancet,* December 13, 1986, 1375; "Draft legislation on infertility services and embryo research," *The Lancet,* December 5, 1987, 1343; "Human embryo research: vote for progress," *The Lancet,* December 5, 1987, 1311; J. Townsend, "Research on human embryos," *The Lancet,* January 3, 1987, 53; "More embryo research?" *Nature,* May 19, 1988, 194; L. Waller, "In Australia, the debate moves to embryo experimentation," *The Hastings Center Report,* June 1987, 21-22; D. Bartels, "Regulating IVF," *Nature,* August 18, 1988, 559-560.

4   D. Brahams, "The hasty British ban on commercial surrogacy," *The Hastings Center Report,* February 1987, 16-19; E. Ross, "Human cloning urged in cell research," Associated Press/AOL News, August 16, 2000.

5   S. Dickman, "West German research agencies oppose new embryo law," *Nature,* May 7, 1987, 6; S. Dickman, "Embryo research ban causes ructions in West Germany," *Nature,* June 30, 1988, 791; S. Dickman, "International outlook for embryo research," *Nature,* June 30, 1988, 6; D. Kirk, "West Germany moving to make IVF a crime," *Science,* July 22, 1988, 406; R. Balling et al., "Moratorium call," *Nature,* August 18, 1988, 560; V. Bolton, P. Braude, and S. Moore, "Ethical bounds," *Nature,* September 29, 1988, 392; C. Coonan, "Germany to protest against human cloning patent," Reuters News Service/America Online, February 23, 2000.

6   L. Silver, *Remaking Eden: How Genetic Engineering and Cloning Will Transform the American Family* (New York: Avon, 1997), 109.

7   As reported by the *Washington Times,* February 10, 2000.

8   S. Begley, "Decoding the human body," *Newsweek,* April 10, 2000, 55.

9   F. Dyson, *The Sun, the Genome, and the Internet: Tools of Scientific Revolution* (New York: Oxford University Press, 1999), 109.

10 R. Gosden, *Designing Babies: The Brave New World of Reproductive Technology* (New York: W. H. Freeman, 1999), 5.

11 Bill Joy, "Why the future doesn't need us," *Wired,* April 2000, 242.

12 Psalm 8:1-5.

13 P. Ramsey, *Fabricated Man* (New Haven, CT: Yale University Press, 1970), 39.

14 Ibid., 38-39, italics mine.

15 For additional information on the current crisis in women's health care and ways to avoid unnecessary treatments, drugs, and surgeries, read: Debra Evans, *The Christian Woman's Guide to Personal Health Care* (Wheaton, IL: Crossway Books, 1999).

16 Psalm 139:13-14.

17 M. Gold, "The baby makers," *Science* 85 (April 1985): 26-38.

18 Psalm 100:3 NASB.

19 G. D. Hodgen, "Pregnancy prevention by intravaginal delivery of a progesterone antagonist: RU486 tampon for menstrual induction and absorption," *Fertility and Sterility* 44 (August 1985): 263-267.

20 N. Tilton and T. Tilton with G. Moore, *Making Miracles* (Garden City, NY: Doubleday & Co., 1985), 156.

21 J. J. Piccone, "This kind of science is best left unused," *USA Today*, March 9, 1989, 6A.

22 "On Human Embryos and Stem Cell Research: An Appeal for Legally and Ethically Responsible Science and Public Policy" was presented at a press conference held on July 1, 1999, on Capitol Hill by four representatives of the group of signers: Nigel Cameron, Ph.D., Advisory Board Chairman, Center for Bioethics and Human Dignity; Frank Young, M.D., Former Commissioner of the U.S. Food and Drug Administration; Edmund Pellegrino, Ph.D., Center for Clinical Bioethics, Georgetown University; and Richard Doerflinger, Associate Director of Policy Development, National Conference of Catholic Bishops. Other signers included C. Everett Koop, M.D., former Surgeon General of the United States; Arthur Dyck, Ph.D., Saltonstall Professor of Population Ethics, Harvard University; C. Christopher Hook, M.D., Director of Ethics Education, Mayo Clinic Graduate School of Medicine; and Dianne Nutwell Irving, former Bench Research Biochemist/Biologist, National Institutes of Health. For more information contact: The Center for Bioethics and Human Dignity, 2065 Half Day Road, Bannockburn, IL 60015 or www.stemcellresearch.org.

23 Sen. Sam Brownback, "The embryo-cell battleground," Op-Ed, August 29, 2000, Infonet-list, 8/30/00, #2242.

24 Cord Blood Registry, 8/28/00, http://www.prnewswire.com.

25 Op. cit.

AFTERWORD

1 C. S. Lewis, *The Abolition of Man* (New York: Macmillan, 1947; 1965), 89.

2 J. Lejeune, in *Ethical Issues in Human Genetics*, Bruce Hilton, et al., ed. (New York: Plenum Press, 1973), p. 113-114.

3 L. Kass, "Implications of Prenatal Diagnosis for the Human Right to Life," in ibid., 188.

4 Ibid., 187.

5 Ibid., 185, 187, 188.

6 Isaiah 45:9-12, *New English Bible*.

7 1 Corinthians 1:20, 27 and 28.

APPENDIX A

1 Pope John Paul II, Discourse to those taking part in the 81st Congress of the Italian

Society of Internal Medicine and the 82nd Congress of the Italian Society of General Surgery, October 27, 1980: AAS 72 (1980) 1126.

2 Pope Paul VI, Discourse to the General Assembly of the United Nations, October 4, 1965: AAS 57 (1965) 878; encyclical *Populorum Progressio*, 13: AAS 59 (1967) 263.

3 Pope Paul VI, Homily during the Mass Closing the Holy Year, December 25, 1975: AAS 68 (1976) 145; Pope John Paul II, encyclical *Dives in Misericordia*, AAS 72 (1980) 1124.

4 Pope John Paul II, Discourse to those taking part in the 35th General Assembly of the World Medical Association, October 29, 1983: AAS 76 (1984) 390.

5 Cf. Declaration *Dignitatis Humanae*, 2.

6 Pastoral constitution *Gaudium et Specs*, 22; Pope John Paul II, encyclical *Redemptor Hominis*, 8: AAS 71 (1979) 270-272.

7 Cf. *Gaudium et Spes*, 35.

8 Ibid., 15; Cf. also *Populorum Progressio*, 20: AAS 59 (1967) 267; *Redemptor Hominis*, 8: AAS 71 (1979) 286-289; Pope John Paul II, apostolic exhortation *Familiaris Consortio*, 8: AAS 74 (1982) 89.

9 *Familiaris Consortio*, 11: AAS 74 (1982) 92.

10 Cf. Pope Paul VI, encyclical *Humanae Vitae*, 10: AAS 60 (1968) 487-488.

11 Pope John Paul II, Discourse to the members of the 35th General Assembly of the World Medical Association, October 29, 1983: AAS 76 (1984) 393.

12 Cf. *Familiaris Consortio*, 11: AAS 74 (1982) 91-92; cf. also *Gaudium et Spes*, 50.

13 Congregation for the Doctrine of the Faith, Declaration on Procured Abortion, 9, AAS 66 (1974) 736-737.

14 Pope John Paul II, Discourse to those taking part in the 35th General Assembly of the World Medical Association, October 29, 1983: AAS 76 (1984) 390.

15 Pope John XXIII, encyclical *Mater et Magistra*, 111: AAS 53 (1961) 447.

16 *Gaudium et Spes*, 24.

17 Cf. Pope Pius XII, encyclical *Humani Generis*: AAS 42 (1950) 575; Pope Paul VI, *Professio Fidei*: AAS 60 (1968) 436.

18 *Mater et Magistra*, III; cf. Pope John Paul II, Discourse to priests participating in a Seminary on "Responsible Procreation," September 17, 1983, *Insegnamenti di Giovanni Paolo II*, VI, 2 (1983) 562: "At the origin of each human person there is a creative act of God: No man comes into existence by chance; he is always the result of the creative love of God."

19 Cf. *Gaudium et Spes*, 24.

20 Cf. Pope Pius XII, Discourse to the St. Luke Medical-Biological Union, November 12, 1944: *Discorsi e Radiomessaggi*, VI (1944-1945) 191-192.

21 Cf, *Gaudium et Spes*, 50.

22 Cf. Ibid., 51: "When it is a question of harmonizing married love with the responsible transmission of life, the moral character of one's behavior does not depend only on the good intention and the evaluation of the motives: The objective criteria must be used, criteria drawn from the nature of the human person and human acts, criteria which respect the total meaning of mutual self-giving and human procreation in the context of true love."

23 *Gaudium et Spes*, 51.

24 Holy See, Charter of the Rights of the Family, 5: *L'Osservatore Romano,* November 25, 1983.

25 Congregation for the Doctrine of the Faith, Declaration on Procured Abortion, 12-13: AAS 66 (1974) 738.

26 Cf. Pope Paul VI, Discourse to participants in the 23rd National Congress of Italian Catholic Jurists, December 9, 1972: AAS 64 (1972) 777.

27 The obligation to avoid disproportionate risks involves an authentic respect for human beings and the uprightness of therapeutic intentions. It implies that the doctor "above all . . . must carefully evaluate the possible negative consequences which the necessary use of a particular exploratory technique may have upon the unborn child and avoid recourse to diagnostic procedures which do not offer sufficient guarantees of their honest purpose and substantial harmlessness. And if, as often happens in human choices, a degree of risk must be undertaken, he will take care to assure that it is justified by a truly urgent need for the diagnosis and by the importance of the results that can be achieved by it for the benefit of the unborn child himself" (Pope John Paul II, Discourse to participants in the Pro-Life Movement Congress, December 3, 1982: *Insegnamenti di Giovanni Paolo II,* V, 3 (1982) 1512. This clarification concerning "proportionate risk" is also to be kept in mind in the following sections of the present Instruction, whenever this terms appears.

28 Pope John Paul II, Discourse to the participants in the 35th General Assembly of the World Medical Association, October 29, 1983: AAS 76 (1984) 392.

29 Cf. Ibid., Address to a meeting of the Pontifical Academy of Sciences, October 23, 1982: AAS 75 (1983) 37: "I condemn, in the most explicit and formal way, experimental manipulations of the human embryo, since the human being, from conception to death, cannot be exploited for any purpose whatsoever."

30 Charter of the Rights of the Family, 4b. *L'Osservatore Romano,* November 25, 1983.

31 Cf. Pope John Paul II, Address to the participants in the Pro-Life Movement Congress, December 3, 1982: *Insegnamenti di Giovanni Paolo II,* V, 3 (1982) 1151: "Any form of experimentation on the fetus that may damage its integrity or worsen its condition is unacceptable, except in the case of a final effort to save it from death." Congregation for the Doctrine of the Faith, Declaration on Euthanasia, 4: AAS 72 (1980) 550: "In the absence of other sufficient remedies, it is permitted, with the patient's consent, to have recourse to the means provided by the most advanced medical techniques, even if these means are still at the experimental stage and are not without a certain risk."

32 No one, before coming into existence, can claim a subjective right to begin to exist; nevertheless, it is legitimate to affirm the right of the child to have a fully human origin through conception in conformity with the personal nature of the human being. Life is a gift that must be bestowed in a manner worthy both of the subject receiving it and of the subjects transmitting it. This statement is to be borne in mind also for what will be explained concerning artificial human procreation.

33 Cf. Pope John Paul II, Discourse to those taking part in the 35th General Assembly of the World Medical Association, October 29, 1983: AAS 76 (1984) 391.

34 Cf. *Gaudium et Spes,* 50.

35 Cf. *Familiaris Consortio,* 14: AAS 74 (1982) 96.

36 Cf. Pope Pius XII, Discourse to those taking part in the Fourth International Congress of Catholic Doctors, September 29, 1949: AAS 41 (1949) 559. According to the plan of the Creator, "a man leaves his father and his mother and cleaves to his wife, and they

become one flesh" (Gn. 2:24). The unity of marriage, bound to the order of creation, is a truth accessible to natural reason. The Church's tradition and magisterium frequently make reference to the Book of Genesis, both directly and through the passages of the New Testament to refer to it: Mt. 19:4-6; Mk 10:5-8; Eph 5:31. Cf. Athenagoras, *Legatio pro christianis*, 33: PG 58 597; St. Leo the Great, *Epist. ad Rusticum*, 4: PL 54, 1204; Innocent III, Epist. *Gaudemus in Domino*: DS 778; Council of Lyons II, IV Session: DS 860; Council of Trent, XXIV Session: DS 1978, 1802; Pope Leo XIII, encyclical *Arcanum Divinae Sapientiae*: AAS 12 (1879-1880) 388-391; Pope Pius XI, encyclical *Casti Connubii*: AAS 22 (1930) 546-547; *Gaudium et Spes*, 48; *Familiaris Consortio*, 19; Code of Canon Law, Canon 1056.

37   Cf. Pope Pius XII, Discourse to those taking part in the Fourth International Congress of Catholic Doctors, September 29, 1949 41 (1949) 560; Discourse to those taking part in the Congress of Italian Catholic Union of Midwives, October 29, 1951: AAS 43 (1951) 850; Code of Canon Law, Canon 1134.

38   *Humanae Vitae*, 12.

39   Ibid.

40   Pope Pius XII, Discourse to those taking part in the Second Naples World Congress on Fertility and Human Sterility, May 19, 1956: AAS 48 (1956) 470.

41   Code of Canon Law, Canon 1061. According to this canon, the conjugal act is that by which the marriage is consummated if the couple "have performed (it) between themselves in a human manner."

42   Cf. *Gaudium et Spes*, 14.

43   Cf. Pope John Paul II, General Audience, January 16, 1980: *Insegnamenti di Giovanni Paolo II*, III, 1 (1980) 148-152.

44   Ibid., Discourse to those taking part in the 35th General Assembly of the World Medical Association, October 29, 1983: AAS 76 (1984) 393.

45   Cf. *Gaudium et Spes*, 51.

46   Ibid., 50.

47   Cf. Pope Pius XII, Discourse to those taking part in the Fourth International Congress of Catholic Doctors, October 29, 1949: AAS 41 (1949) 560: "It would be erroneous . . . to think that the possibility of resorting to this means (artificial fertilization) might render valid a marriage between persons unable to contract it because of the "impedimentum impotentiae."

48   A similar question was dealt with by Pope Paul VI, *Humanae Vitae*, 14.

49   Cf. supra: I, 1ff.

50   *Familiaris Consortio*, 14: AAS 74 (1982) 96.

51   Cf. Response to the Holy Office, March 17, 1897: DS 3323; Pope Pius XII, Discourse to those taking part in the Fourth International Congress of Catholic Doctors, September 29, 1949: AAS 41 (1949) 560; Discourse to the Italian Catholic Union of Midwives, October 29, 1951: AAS 43 (1951) 850; Discourse to those taking part in the Second Naples World Congress on Fertility and Human Sterility, May 19, 1956: AAS, 48 (1956) 471-473; Discourse to those taking part in the Seventh International Congress of the International Society of Hematology, September 1958: AAS 50 (1958) 733; *Mater et Magistra*, III.

52   Pope Pius XII, Discourse to the Italian Catholic Union of Midwives, October 29, 1951: AAS 43 (1951) 850.

53 Ibid., Discourse to those taking part in the Fourth International Congress of Catholic Doctors, September 29, 1949; AAS 41 (1949) 560.

54 Congregation for the Doctrine of the Faith, Declaration on Certain Questions Concerning Sexual Ethics, 9: AAS 68 (1976) 86, which quotes *Gaudium et Spes,* 51. Cf. Decree of the Holy Office, August 2, 1919: AAS 21 (1929) 490: Pope Pius XII, Discourse to those taking part in the 26th Congress of the Italian Society of Urology, October 8, 1953: AAS 45 (1953) 678.

55 Cf. Pope John XXIII, *Mater et Magistra,* III.

56 Cf. Pope Pius XII, Discourse to those taking part in the Fourth International Congress of Catholic Doctors, September 29, 1949: AAS 41 (1949), 560.

57 Cf. Ibid., Discourse to those taking part in the Second Naples World Congress on Fertility and Human Sterility, May 19, 1956: AAS 48 (1956) 471-473.

58 *Familiaris Consortio,* 14: AAS 74 (1982) 97.

59 Cf. *Dignitatis Humanae,* 7.

APPENDIX B

1 "Guest editorial: finding the truth in birth—a leap of faith," *International Journal of Childbirth Education* 4 (February 1989): 20.

 2 "Christian Tradition and the Control of Reproduction," in L. J. Nelson, ed., *The Death Decision* (Ann Arbor, MI: Servant Books, 1984), 15.

GLOSSARY

abortifacient: Any drug or substance capable of inducing an abortion.

abortion: The spontaneous or deliberate ending of a pregnancy before the developing baby can survive outside the mother's womb.

abortion rate: The number of abortions during a specific time in relation to the total number of women between the ages of fifteen and forty-four in a given population. (Usually expressed as the number of abortions per 1,000 women ages fifteen to forty-four.)

acrosome: The lead end of the head of a sperm that releases enzymes to dissolve the surface of the ovum.

adhesion: A holding together by new connective tissue of two structures that are normally separate, produced by inflammation, surgery, or injury.

alphafetoprotein [AFP] test: Maternal blood test routinely performed during pregnancy to diagnose neural tube defects such as spina bifida and anencephaly.

American College of Obstetricians and Gynecologists [ACOG]: National organization of certified specialists in obstetrics and gynecology.

amniocentesis: Diagnostic sampling of amniotic fluid during pregnancy, especially for the purpose of genetic analysis. The fluid is obtained by puncturing the mother's abdomen and womb with a special needle.

amnion: The fluid-filled sac or membrane enclosing the developing baby within the womb; also referred to as the "bag of waters."

amniotic fluid: A colorless liquid surrounding the baby within the womb.

amniotomy: The artificial rupture of the amniotic sac by a physician.

anesthesia: The partial or complete loss of sensation with or without loss of consciousness as a result of injury, disease, or the administration of a drug or gas.

anovulation: The absence of ovulation.

antenatal: Occurring just before birth.

antepartum: Around the time of birth; a term used to describe the labor and delivery functions and staff of a hospital.

artificial embryonation [AE]: The process by which a human ovum is artificially inseminated within a woman's reproductive tract and then flushed out five to seven days later for transfer to another woman's womb; the transfer of an embryo from the womb of a fertile donor to the uterus of an infertile recipient who will attempt to carry the embryo to term. Also called *in vivo fertilization* and *surrogate embryo transfer* [SET].

artificial insemination [AI]: Semen deposited in the vagina by a mechanical instrument rather than a man's penis.

artificial insemination by donor [AID]: Artificial insemination using sperm obtained from a donor.

artificial insemination by husband[AIH]: Artificial insemination using sperm obtained from one's husband.

artificial placentation: The mechanical provision of nutrients and removal of waste products from a fetus.

artificial placentation system [APS]: A set of interrelated devices that function as an artificial placenta.

artificial womb: A man-made device designed for conducting gestation outside the human body.

aspermia: The absence of sperm and semen.

azoospermia: The absence of sperm in semen.

basal body temperature: The temperature of the body—taken orally, rectally, or vaginally—after at least three hours of sleep, taken before rising.

Basal Body Temperature method of family planning [BBT]: A method of family planning that relies on identifying the fertile period of a woman's menstrual cycle for the purpose of attempting or avoiding pregnancy.

biopsy: The surgical removal of a sample of tissue for diagnostic purposes.

birth: The process by which a new human being enters the world and begins life outside the mother's body.

birth center: A facility designed to prevent interference in the natural process of childbirth—may be freestanding or connected to a hospital. Many obstetrical departments are now naming redesigned in-hospital units "birthing centers" for consumer appeal. If continuous electronic fetal monitoring, induction of labor, artificial rupture of the membranes, epidural anesthesia, and routine episiotomies are frequently being conducted in a facility using this name, it is *not* a birth center—it is a *hospital*.

birth control: The prevention of birth.

birth mother: A woman who conceives a child as a result of sexual intercourse or artificial insemination and places her child in a family by adoption at the time of birth.

birth rate: The number of births during a specific period of time in relation to the total population of a certain area.

blastocyst: The fertilized ovum during its second week of development; the name means "many-celled hollow ball."

bonding: The deepening of intimacy over time between two people through emotional, physical, and spiritual interactions. Touch, eye contact, speech, and loving gestures create, sustain, and magnify human bonds within the family.

cannula: A hollow tube or sheath.

catheter: A thin plastic tube designed to perform invasive medical procedures upon the body.

certified nurse-midwife [C.N.M.]: A registered nurse who is a graduate of an approved training program and who has passed a certification examination.

cervix: The fixed, neck-like segment of the lower uterus that forms the passageway into the vagina.

cesarean section: The surgical removal of a baby through an incision in the mother's abdominal tissue and uterine wall.

chlamydia: A generic term for infection caused by the organism *chlamydia trichomonas*; a sexually transmitted disease characterized by a thick yellow discharge from the cervix that may result in pelvic abscesses, pelvic inflammatory disease, and involuntary sterility. Also called *mucopurulent cervicitis*.

chorion: The outermost membrane covering the developing baby during the first trimester. The chorion encloses the amnion, lies closest to the wall of the uterus, and eventually becomes the placenta.

chorionic villi: Tiny projections extending from the surface of the chorion that secrete human chorionic gonadotropin [HCG].

chorionic villi sampling [CVS]: Diagnostic test using chorionic villi tissue for the purpose of genetic analysis during the first trimester of pregnancy. CVS is performed by a physician using ultrasound as a guide to pass a catheter through the vagina and cervix into the womb to the chorion. A few cells from the chorionic surface are removed by suction and then examined for chromosomal abnormalities, certain genetic conditions, and fetal sex.

chromosome: Threadlike bodies within the nucleus of every cell that make up strands of DNA. These structures contain the genetic material that is passed from parents to their children. Each normal human cell contains forty-six chromosomes arranged in twenty-three pairs from the time of conception.

cilia: Hairlike filaments lining the inner wall of the fallopian tubes. These filaments beat rhythmically to create a current that takes the egg toward the uterus.

clomiphene citrate [Clomid, Serophene]: A drug used to induce ovulation in anovulatory women. Its precise mechanism of action is unknown.

conception: The fertilization of the egg by a sperm that initiates the growth of a human being and triggers the onset of pregnancy. The American College of Obstetricians and Gynecologists, however, changed the definition of conception in September 1965: "Fertilization is the *union* of the spermatozoan and ovum; conception is the *implantation* of the fertilized ovum." (ACOG Terminology Bulletin No. 1) This allows birth control methods that prevent implantation of fertilized ova to be called contraceptives rather than contragestives or abortifacients.

conceptus: Fertilized ovum or "pre-embryo"; term used by researchers to dehumanize the earliest stages of human development following conception.

contraception: The act of preventing conception.

contraceptive: Any drug, device, surgery, or method of family planning that prevents conception.

contragestive: Any drug, device, or surgery that interrupts pregnancy and induces an abortion.

corpus luteum: The temporary gland created within a ruptured ovarian follicle; secretes hormones to protect and maintain pregnancy until the placenta matures and takes over this role. The name means "yellow body."

cryobank: Place where frozen sperm is stored; a commercial business selling frozen sperm.

cryopreservation: The storage of living cells by the use of special chemicals and ultra- rapid freezing.

cystic fibrosis: A disease of infants, children, adolescents, and young adults affecting the sweat and mucus-secreting glands, resulting in chronic lung disease, pancreatic insufficiency, abnormally salty sweat, and, in some cases, liver disease.

diethylstilbestrol [DES]: A synthetic estrogen used during the 1950s and 1960s to prevent miscarriage. In 1971 it was found to cause a rare form of vaginal cancer, and vaginal changes were found in a significant number of the daughters born to women who had taken DES during pregnancy.

dilation: The process of opening. In labor, uterine contractions press the baby against the cervix to open the womb. In gynecological procedures, metal rods of increasing size are inserted into the cervix to stretch it open. In either case, cervical dilation is accompanied by a menstrual-like cramping sensation.

dilation and curettage [D&C]: Name literally means "opening, cutting, and scraping." A surgical procedure in which the cervix is forcibly opened, and the inside of the uterus is scraped with a sharp, spoonlike instrument called a curette. The procedure is used to remove polyps or an overgrowth of uterine tissue as a way of diagnosing cancer or after childbirth to remove tissue retained in the womb. This is also a method of abortion involving the dismemberment of the developing child by suction and its extraction from the uterus.

dilation and evacuation [D&E]: A surgical procedure used to abort a child during the second trimester of pregnancy, requiring crushing of the skull and surgical dismemberment of the baby's body before removal from the womb.

DNA: Deoxyribonucleic acid—a complex molecule carrying genetic information within the nucleus of a cell.

DNA probe: A specific DNA sequence used to identify a like sequence in genetic diagnosis.

donor egg: An egg given up by its biological mother to another woman or couple. The donor's ovum unites with the infertile woman's husband's sperm. The baby is nurtured within the adoptive mother's uterus during pregnancy.

donor embryo: A baby in the earliest stage of human development. It is produced by gametes uniting in a glass dish or within the genetic mother's reproductive tract. The embryo is transferred to a different woman's womb for gestation.

ectopic pregnancy: A pregnancy occurring outside the uterus, usually in a fallopian tube.

ejaculation: The sudden release of semen from the male urethra.

egg donor: A woman who gives or sells her eggs to another woman.

embryo donor: A woman who gives or sells her embryo to another woman.

embryo: In humans, an unborn child before the eighth week of pregnancy—a period that involves rapid growth, initial development of the major organ systems, and early formation of the main external features.

embryo transfer [ET]: The placement of an embryo into a woman's uterus. The embryo being transferred may have been fertilized *in vitro* (within the laboratory) or *in vivo* (within the reproductive tract of an egg donor).

embryo transplant: The placement of a donated or purchased embryo into a gestational (surrogate) mother's uterus.

endocrine system The system of glands within the body, including the thymus, pituitary, parathyroid, thyroid, adrenals, ovaries (in females), and testicles (in males).

endocrinologist: A physician specializing in diseases of the endocrine system.

endocrinology/infertility: The branch of obstetrics and gynecology dealing with the hormones, diseases, and conditions that affect fertility.

endometriosis: A growth of endometrial tissue outside the uterus, thought to occur in about 15 percent of women. Women who do not get pregnant until later in life are more likely to acquire this disease, with the average age of diagnosis being thirty-seven. Pregnancy seems to prevent or delay the onset of this problem. The most common symptoms of endometriosis are severe menstrual cramps, painful intercourse, painful bowel movements, and soreness above the pubic bones. Endometriosis is a factor in many cases of female infertility.

endometrium: The inner lining of the uterus.

endorphin: Any one of the substances of the nervous system made by the pituitary gland producing morphine-like effects as a way of reducing pain within the body.

epidemic: A disease spread rapidly throughout the population.

estrogen: A hormone secreted by the ovaries that regulates the development of secondary sexual characteristics in women and produces cyclic changes in tissue lining the vagina and the uterus. Natural estrogens include estradiol, estrone, and their metabolic product, estriol. When used therapeutically, estrogens are usually given in a conjugated form, such as ethinyl estradiol, conjugated estrogens (USP), or the synthetic estrogen DES (diethylstilbestrol).

ethics: A system of moral principles or standards governing conduct.

eugenic abortion: The deliberate killing of a preborn child for eugenic reasons.

eugenics: The science that deals with the physical, moral, and intellectual improvement of the human race through genetic control. *Negative eugenics* includes those measures that seek to restrict the numbers of offspring with genetically undesirable traits; *positive eugenics* includes those measures that seek to bring about an increase in the numbers of offspring of families with genetically desirable traits. Eugenics is based upon Darwinian, or evolutionary, theory.

extracorporeal membrane oxygenation[ECMO]: The mechanical exchange of oxygen, waste products, and nutrients on behalf of a baby incapable of breathing; the artificial accomplishment of placental function outside the mother's body.

evolution: The theory proposed by Charles Darwin that the composition of all living matter is formed in response to environmental conditions. Any changes provoked, however, do not depend solely on the environment but upon the interaction of an organism with its environment. Thus organisms may or may not respond to the environment by *adaptive genetic change*. This belief concludes that failure to respond positively to the environment may lead to diminution and eventually extinction of a species; successful biologic responses enable the species to survive and expand. Evolution theory leads to three conclusions about the human species: 1.) As a species, human beings are in a process of development; therefore, no finished life form exists, including human life. 2.) Chance plays a major role in biological change—chance genetic variation leading to diversity within a species and chance environmental changes; natural selection integrates these two components to produce biological change. 3.) Competition for survival exists between species and within a species, characterized by a fierce struggle that results in the triumph of the biologically superior over the inferior. These tenets place human identity on a developmental continuum rather than upon an absolute or fixed position of value within nature.

fallopian tube: The duct that conveys the egg from the ovary to the womb.

family physician: A physician who has completed a three-year residency in family practice medicine.

fertilization: see *conception*.

fertile: Having the ability to conceive and bear offspring; fruitful; not sterile.

fertile mucus: A substance secreted by the cervix that is capable of facilitating the transport of sperm through a woman's reproductive tract.

fertile period: The time during the menstrual cycle in which conception may take place, beginning three to six days before ovulation and ending two to three days afterward.

fetus: The term applied to a developing baby after the eighth week of pregnancy until birth.

fibroid: A noncancerous tumor of the uterus, usually occurring in women thirty to fifty years of age.

fimbria: The fringelike borders of the open ends of the fallopian tubes.

follicle: A pouchlike recessed structure in the ovary containing an immature ovum called an oocyte and the cells surrounding the oocyte.

follicle-stimulating hormone [FSH]: A hormone secreted by the pituitary gland that is responsible for stimulating the growth of ovarian follicles in women and the development of sperm (spermatogenesis) in men.

forceps: An instrument with two blades and handles designed to forcibly pull the baby, usually by the head, from the vagina.

FSH: See *follicle stimulating hormone.*

gamete: A mature male or female reproductive cell; the spermatozoon or ovum.

gamete intrafallopian transfer [GIFT]: The placement of sperm and oocytes into an unblocked fallopian tube through a laparoscope for *in vivo* fertilization.

gender: The specific sex of a person; male or female.

gene: The basic unit of heredity in a chromosome that carries characteristics from parent to child.

general anesthesia: Medically induced loss of feeling and sensation, including the loss of memory and consciousness.

generation: The act or process of reproduction; procreation.

genesis: Origin; generation; the act of producing or procreating.

genetic code: A code that fixes amino acids, building blocks of body tissue proteins, into patterns that determine the traits of offspring.

genetic diagnosis: Analysis of an individual's chromosomal makeup for the purpose of identifying a genetic disorder.

genetic engineering: The process of making new DNA molecules.

geneticist: A specialist in genetics.

genetics: The science of heredity and its variations; the study of resemblances and differences of related organisms resulting from the interaction of their genes and the environment.

genic: Of or resembling a gene or genes.

gestation: The period between conception and birth.

gestational mother: See *surrogate mother.*

genome: The complete set of genetic instructions carried within the DNA molecule.

genotype: The unique genetic constitution of a specific person or organism.

gonadotropin: A hormone capable of stimulating the gonads, or primary sex organs.

gonorrhea: A specific, contagious inflammatory infection of the genital mucus membrane, mouth, or anus of either sex transmitted by intimate sexual contact.

gynecologist: A physician who specializes in the problems of the female sexual organs.

gynecology: The branch of medicine dealing with diseases and problems of the female reproductive tract.

gyne-, gyno-: Prefix meaning woman, female.

gynetech: A new form of medicine specializing in the technological control of human reproduction.

hamster-egg penetration assay: Diagnostic test in which sperm are incubated with hamster eggs to test their capability to fertilize ova.

HCG: See *human chorionic gonadotropin.*

HMG: See *human menopausal gonadotropin.*

healing: The process or act in which health is restored to the body, emotions, mind, or spirit.

health: A state of physical, emotional, mental, and spiritual well-being.

heterologous insemination: See *artificial insemination by donor.*

homologous insemination: See *artificial insemination by husband.*

high-risk pregnancy: Term describing the probability that complications during pregnancy and childbirth may occur.

home birth: Birth taking place at home. As used by those who advocate home birth for healthy childbearing women, the term indicates a planned home birth attended by skilled maternity care providers. As used by those seeking to eliminate home birth, the term is used to indicate all births taking place outside the hospital, including miscarriages, early arrivals during transport, unattended and unplanned home births, and involuntary home births among women too poor to afford hospitalization.

hormone: Chemical substances, produced by ductless glands in one part of the body, that affect an organ or group of cells in another area of the body.

hospital birth: Birth taking place in a hospital.

human chorionic gonadotropin [HCG]: A hormone produced by the chorionic villi that is responsible for triggering the release of progesterone and estrogen, measured during a pregnancy test through urine. HCG is extracted from the urine of pregnant women and administered by injection to stimulate ovarian and testicular function.

human menopausal gonadotropin [HMG]: A hormone extracted from the urine of postmenopausal women that can be administered by injection to stimulate the ovaries and testes.

hyster-, hystero-: Prefix—womb; hysteria.

hysterectomy: The surgical removal of the uterus.

hystero-oophorectomy: The surgical removal of the uterus and one or both ovaries.

hysterosalpingogram: X-ray study of the uterus and fallopian tubes after injecting radiopaque material into these organs; used for diagnosis of infertility or sterility.

hysterosalpingo-oophorectomy: The surgical removal of the uterus, fallopian tubes, and ovaries.

hysteroscopy: Inspection of the inside of the uterus by means of a lighted instrument called a hysteroscope.

hysterotomy: 1. Incision of the uterus. 2. Cesarean section. 3. A method of induced abortion conducted through incisions in the mother's abdominal wall and uterus.

iatrogenic: Produced or caused by a physician.

idiopathic infertility: Infertility of unknown cause.

implantation: Embedding of the developing baby in the lining of the uterus.

induced abortion: An intentional termination of a pregnancy before an unborn child has developed to the point where he or she can survive outside the uterus.

induction of labor: The artificial production of labor.

infertile: The inability to conceive or produce offspring.

infertility: The state of being infertile or unable to carry a pregnancy. Medically defined as the inability of a couple to conceive after twelve months of intercourse without contraception.

intrauterine contraceptive device [IUCD]: A form of contraception consisting of inserting a bent strip of plastic or copper into the uterus to prevent pregnancy. The device does not prevent ovulation or conception.

IUD: See *intrauterine contraceptive device.*

IVF/ET: See *in vitro fertilization* and *embryo transfer.*

invasive techniques: Any medical procedure that penetrates the boundaries of the body.

in vitro fertilization [IVF]: Conception occurring in laboratory apparatus. The name literally means "in glass" fertilization.

in vivo fertilization: Fertilization within the human body.

labor: The series of stages during the process of childbirth through which the baby is born and the uterus returns to a normal state; contractions of the uterus that result in the birth of a baby.

lactation: The process by which milk is produced and secreted by the breasts for nourishing an infant.

laminaria: Kelp or seaweed which, when dried, is capable of absorbing water and expanding with considerable force; used to dilate the cervical canal prior to a surgical abortion.

laparoscopy: Exploration of the pelvic cavity by means of a lighted instrument called a laparoscope.

laparotomy: The surgical opening of the abdomen; an abdominal operation.

laser: Acronym for *light amplification by stimulated emission of radiation.*

laser surgery: Any operative procedure that employs a laser rather than a scalpel to excise body tissue.

lay midwife: A birth attendant who has acquired her skills through apprenticeship and experience rather than formalized schooling.

liable: To be legally responsible.

litigate: To seek remedy through a court of law, including the act of carrying on a lawsuit, by means of presenting evidence of damage or harm.

low-risk pregnancy: Term used to describe the probability that pregnancy and childbirth will be normal and uneventful.

luteal: Referring to the corpus luteum, its functions or its effects.

luteinizing hormone [LH]: A hormone produced by the pituitary gland in both males and females. It stimulates the production of testosterone in men and the secretion of estrogen in women.

malpractice, medical: The failure of a health-care professional to render proper services through reprehensible ignorance, negligence, or criminal intent toward a client; bad, wrong, or injudicious treatment resulting in injury, unnecessary suffering, or death; the misconduct or misuse of medicine.

menarche: The onset of menstruation; the beginning of the first menstrual cycle.

menopause: The end of menstruation when the menses stop as a normal result of the decline of monthly hormonal cycles.

menotropin [Pergonal]: See *human menopausal gonadotropin*.

menstrual cycle: The cycle of hormonal changes that begins at puberty and repeats itself on a monthly basis unless interrupted by pregnancy, lactation, medication, or metabolic disorders.

menstruation: The natural process by which the lining of the non-pregnant uterus is cast off, resulting in a discharge of blood and mucosal tissue from the vagina.

menstrual extraction: Removal of the lining of the uterus by suction before menstruation occurs; also a method of induced abortion.

microsurgery: Surgery performed while a physician observes through a microscope.

midwife: A birth attendant who respects nature while supporting and supervising the natural processes of labor during childbirth; a woman who practices the art of midwifery.

midwifery: The traditional practice of providing help and assistance to women during childbirth, characterized by watching and waiting upon nature's design for labor.

miscarriage: The spontaneous loss of a baby before the twenty-eighth week of pregnancy.

monogamy: The practice of marrying only once for life.

morbidity: A state of illness or disease.

morning-after pill: A very large dose of estrogen taken orally within twenty-four to seventy-two hours after intercourse to terminate a pregnancy.

mortality: Death.

mortality rate: The number of deaths during a specific time within a given population. When dealing with fetuses and babies, the rate is based on number of deaths per 1,000 live births; when considering mothers, the rate quoted represents the number of deaths per 100,000 pregnancies.

mucus: The slippery, sticky secretion released by mucous membranes and glands.

natal: Referring to birth.

Natural Family Planning [NFP]: Any method of family planning that does not use drugs or devices to prevent conception.

neonate: A newborn baby; a baby less than twenty-eight days old.

neonatologist: A pediatrician specializing in the care of newborn babies.

neural tube: Tube formed from fusion of the neural folds from which the brain and spinal cord arise.

neural tube defect: A condition resulting from the failure of the neural tube to close during fetal development, resulting in spina bifida or anencephaly.

noninvasive: Referring to any test, treatment, or procedure that does not penetrate the boundaries of the body.

nurse-midwife: See *certified nurse-midwife.*

obstetrics: The branch of medicine dealing with the management of pregnancy and childbirth.

oligogenics: The limitation of offspring through utilizing some form of birth control.

oligospermia: Deficient levels of sperm in seminal fluid; the condition may be temporary or permanent.

oocyte: The early or primitive human egg before it has completed development.

oogenesis: The growth and development of female eggs.

oophorectomy: The surgical removal of an ovary.

oral contraceptive: A steroid drug taken to induce temporary infertility.

orchiectomy: The surgical removal of a testicle.

osteoporosis: Increased porosity of bone tissue; the loss of normal bone density marked by a thinning of bone tissue and the growth of small openings in the bone.

ova: Human eggs; female reproductive or germ cells; a cell capable of developing into a new organism of the same species. (Singular: *ovum.*)

ovary: One of the pair of primary sexual organs in females located on each side of the lower abdomen beside the uterus. The ovaries produce the reproductive cell, or ovum, and two known hormones, estrogen and progesterone.

ovariectomy: The removal of an ovary or a portion of the ovary.

oviduct: See *fallopian tube.*

Ovulation Method of family planning [OM]: A method of family planning that relies on the observation of the type and amount of cervical mucus secreted during the menstrual cycle as a means of predicting fertility.

ovum donor: See *egg donor*.

ovum transfer [OT]: See *embryo transfer*.

pelvic inflammatory disease [PID]: Inflammation of the female reproductive organs in the pelvis, often resulting in scarring, blocked fallopian tubes, and infertility.

pelvic floor: The muscles and tissues that form the base of the pelvis.

pelvis: The bowl-shaped lower portion of the trunk of the body.

perinatal: The period from the twenty-eighth week of pregnancy to one week after the baby's birth.

perinatologist: A physician who specializes in maternal-fetal medicine.

perineum: The part of the body lying between the inner thighs, with the buttocks to the rear and the genitals to the front.

placenta: A temporary organ created to exchange waste products and carry nutrients between mother and baby during pregnancy. The placenta produces hormones to protect and maintain gestation.

polyp: A small, tumorlike growth that protrudes from a mucous membrane surface.

postcoital test: Samples of deposited semen and vaginal-cervical discharge removed from different areas along the length of the cervical canal for diagnostic analysis; the microscopic analysis of vaginal and cervical secretions within several hours of sexual intercourse.

postpartum: After childbirth.

pregnancy: The growth and development of a new person inside a woman's uterus.

premenstrual syndrome [PMS]: The presence of a set of interrelated symptoms that recur regularly during the same phase of each menstrual cycle.

prenatal: The period before birth.

progesterone: Hormone produced by the corpus luteum and, during pregnancy, the placenta; this hormone prepares the uterine lining for implantation and the breasts for lactation and relaxes smooth muscle to prevent uterine contractions and subsequent pregnancy loss.

progestin: Any one of a group of hormones, natural or synthetic, that have progesterone-like effects on the reproductive system.

progestogen: See *progestin*.

prostaglandins: A group of strong hormone-like fatty acids that act on certain body organs. Used as a method of inducing labor and terminating pregnancy.

reproductive endocrinologist: An obstetrician-gynecologist who specializes in diagnosing and treating infertility.

RU486: A drug capable of inducing abortion by inhibiting the secretion of progesterone.

semen: The thick, white-colored fluid released by the male sex organs for the purpose of transporting sperm.

seminal fluid: See *semen*.

sex-linked: A genetic characteristic controlled by genes in sex chromosomes.

sexually transmitted disease [STD]: A contagious disease spread through intimate sexual contact.

sexually transmitted infertility: The inability to conceive or produce children as a result of damage to the reproductive organs due to a sexually transmitted disease.

side effect: A reaction resulting from medical treatment or therapy.

sperm: The male cell of reproduction, also called a *spermatozoa* or *gamete*.

sperm antibody test: Antibodies to sperm may be present in a woman's vaginal secretions; this test examines the sperm-mucus interaction.

spermatogenesis: The process of sperm production.

spermatozoon: The mature male sex or germ cells formed within the seminiferous tubules of the testes. (Singular: *spermatozoa.*)

sperm bank: See *cryobank.*

sperm count: An estimate of the number of sperm in a given sample of seminal fluid.

sperm donor: A man who produces sperm through masturbation for use in artificial insemination, usually for a fee.

spermicide: Any chemical substance that kills sperm cells.

sperm motility: The rate at which sperm move from one point to another.

spina bifida: A congenital defect in the walls of the spinal canal, caused by lack of union between the vetebral membranes. The opening exposes the spinal nerves and often results in paralysis.

sterile: The inability to produce children.

sterilization: An act or process that renders a person incapable of reproduction.

stress: Any factor that requires a response or change on the part of an organism or an individual.

stressor: Anything capable of causing wear and tear on the body's mental, physical, emotional, or spiritual resources.

surrogate embryo transfer [SET]: See *artificial embryonation.*

surrogate mother: A woman who agrees to have another couple's embryo transferred to her uterus for the period of gestation until the time of birth; a woman who bears no genetic relationship to the baby in her womb. Common usage: a woman who agrees to be artificially inseminated with the sperm of an infertile woman's husband and to carry the baby until birth for a fee.

symptom: Something felt or noticed by an individual that can be used to detect what is going on within the body.

Sympto-thermal Method of family planning: A method seeking to discern fertility awareness based on the ovulation and basal body temperature methods of family planning.

syphilis: A sexually transmitted disease caused by an organism called a spirochete.

teaching hospital: A hospital associated with a medical institution in which students train and also work with patients.

technician: A person skilled in a particular technique.

technique: The body of specialized procedures and methods used in any particular field.

technological, technology, high-tech: The branch of knowledge that deals with industrial arts, applied science, and engineering; a technological process, invention, method, or the like; in obstetrics and gynecology, medical care characterized by the use of invasive techniques and man-made interventions.

testecotomy: The surgical removal of a testicle. Also called *castration*.

testes: The two male reproductive glands located in the scrotum that produce sperm and the male sex hormone testosterone. (Singular: *testicle* or *testis*.)

testosterone: A naturally secreted hormone in both males and females that is capable of producing masculine secondary sexual characteristics.

therapy: The treatment of an abnormal condition.

thromboembolism: A condition in which a blood vessel is blocked by a clot.

trimester: Period of three months; one of the three phases of pregnancy.

trophoblast: A strand of single cells ringing the blastocyst that will later become the placenta.

tubal cautery: Sterilization of a woman by burning both fallopian tubes.

tubal ligation: Sterilization of a woman via surgical removal of a small segment of each fallopian tube.

tubal pregnancy: A pregnancy in which the early embryo implants within the fallopian tube and cannot develop normally.

ultrasonography: Inaudible high-frequency sound waves used to outline the shape of body organs or a developing baby.

ultrasound: See *ultrasonography*.

urethra: The canal that carries urine from the bladder.

urinary stress incontinence: The involuntary passage of urine when coughing, sneezing, or laughing, resulting from poor sphincter control of the urethra.

urology: The branch of medicine concerned with the care of the urinary tract in men and women and of the male genital tract.

uterine lavage: Flushing of the uterus performed by use of a catheter inserted into the cervix.

uterus: The thick-walled, hollow, muscular female organ of reproduction.

vacuum aspiration: A method of inducing abortion using a suction machine to remove the developing baby, placenta, and amniotic sac from the uterus.

vacuum extractor: An instrument that adheres to the baby's scalp and forcibly pulls the baby out of the birth canal; used as an alternative to forceps.

vagina: The muscular, tubelike membrane that forms the passageway between the uterus and genital entrance. It receives the penis during lovemaking and becomes the canal through which the baby passes during childbirth.

vas deferens: One of a pair of tubes within the male reproductive tract through which sperm pass.

vasectomy: A surgical procedure that produces male sterility by cutting a section out of each vas deferens.

viable: Capable of living, growing, and developing; a baby capable of living outside the uterus.

womb: See *uterus*.

wrongful life action: A lawsuit brought against a physician or health facility because an unwanted child was born.

X-chromosome: The sex-determining chromosome carried by all ova and approximately one-half of sperm.

Y-chromosome: The sex-determining chromosome carried by about one-half of all sperm, never by an egg, that produces a male child.

zygote: The developing egg between the time of fertilization and implantation in the wall of the uterus.

SELECTED READING LIST

Among the many books and articles I read while researching emerging trends in science, technology, eugenics, and reproductive medicine, those listed here stand out from the rest. I owe their authors, regardless of whether I agree with them, a debt of gratitude.

Books

Bonhoeffer, Dietrich, *Ethics* (New York: Macmillan, 1955 [1975]).

Bopp, James, ed., *Human Life and Health Care Ethics* (Frederick, MD: University Publications of America, 1985).

Burtchaell, James, *Rachel Weeping* (New York: Harper & Row, 1982).

Dyson, Freeman, *The Sun, the Genome, and the Internet* (New York: Oxford University Press, 1999).

Edwards, Robert, and Patrick Steptoe, *A Matter of Life* (New York: William Morrow, 1980).

Ellul, Jacques, *The Technological Society* (New York: Alfred A. Knopf, Vintage Books Edition, 1964).

Francoeur, Robert T., *Utopian Motherhood: New Trends in Human Reproduction* (Garden City, NY: Doubleday, 1970).

Gilder, George, *Men and Marriage* (Gretna, LA: Pelican Publishing, 1986).

Godsen, Roger, *Designing Babies* (New York: W. H. Freeman, 1999).

Hamilton, Michael, ed., *The New Genetics and the Future of Man* (Grand Rapids, MI: William B. Eerdmans, 1971).

Hilton, Bruce, Daniel Callahan, Maureen Harris, Peter Condliffe, and Burton Berkley, eds., *Ethical Issues in Human Genetics* (New York, Plenum, 1973).

Iglesias, Teresa, *A Basic Ethic for Man's Well-being: Conscience and the New Scientific Possibilities* (Southport, Merseyside, GB: Gowland & Co., 1989).

Kass, Leon R., *Toward a More Natural Science: Biology and Human Affairs* (New York: The Free Press, 1985).

Kelves, Daniel, *In the Name of Eugenics* (New York: Knopf, 1985).

Kirkendall, Lester A., and Arthur E. Gravatt, eds., *Marriage and Family in the Year 2020* (New York: Prometheus, 1984).

Lewis, C. S., *That Hideous Strength* (New York: Macmillan, 1965).

_____, *The Abolition of Man* (New York: Macmillan, 1965).

McGee, Glenn, ed., *The Human Cloning Debate* (Berkeley, CA: Berkeley Hills Books, 1998).

Ramsey, Paul, *Fabricated Man* (New Haven, CT: Yale University Press, 1970).

Rosenfeld, Albert, *The Second Genesis: The Coming Control of Life* (Englewood Cliffs, NJ: Prentice-Hall, 1969).

Rostand, Jean, *Can Man Be Modified?* (New York: Basic Books, 1959).

Schaeffer, Francis, and C. Everett Koop, *Whatever Happened to the Human Race?* (Wheaton, IL: Crossway Books, 1983).

Silver, Lee, *Remaking Eden: How Genetic Engineering and Cloning Will Transform the American Family* (New York: Avon, 1997).

Articles

Alexander, Leo, "Medical science under dictatorship," *New England Journal of Medicine*, July 14, 1949 ("must" reading for anyone concerned about the devastating impact of utilitarian medicine on civilization and society).

Andrews, Lori B., "Yours, mine and theirs," *Psychology Today*, December 1984.

Annas, George, "Making babies without sex: the law and the profits," *American Journal of Public Health*, 1984.

Ausubel, Frederick, Jon Beckwith, and Karen Janssen, "The politics of genetic engineering: who decides who's defective?" *Psychology Today*, June 1974.

Bolton, Virginia, Peter Braude, and Stephen Moore, "Ethical bounds," *Nature*, September 29, 1988.

Blumberg, Lisa, "The right to live: disability is not a crime," *The Exceptional Parent*, December 1984.

Callahan, Sidney, "Lovemaking and babymaking," *Commonweal*, April 24, 1987.

Chargaff, Erwin, "Engineering a molecular nightmare," *Nature*, May 21, 1987.

Cohen, Libby G., "Selective abortion and the diagnosis of fetal damage: issues and concerns," *Journal of the Association for Persons with Severe Handicaps*, 1986.

Cowley, Geoffrey, "Made to order babies," *Newsweek*, (Special Issue) Winter/Spring 1990.

Edwards, Robert G., "Studies in human conception," *American Journal of Obstetrics and Gynecology*, November 1, 1973.

Edwards, Robert G., and M. Puxon, "Parental consent over embryos," *Nature*, July 19, 1984.

Edwards, Robert G., and David J. Sharpe, "Social values and research in human embryology," *Nature*, May 14, 1971.

Fiedler, Leslie A., "The tyranny of the normal," *The Hastings Center Report*, April 1984.

Fleming, Anne Taylor, "New frontiers in conception," *New York Times Magazine*, July 20, 1980.

Frankel, Charles, "The specter of eugenics," *Commentary*, March 1974.

Johnson, Mary, "Life unworthy of life," *The Disability Rag*, January/February, 1987.

Joy, Bill, "Why the future doesn't need us," *Wired*, April 2000.

Kass, Leon R., "Babies by in vitro fertilization: unethical experiments on the unborn?" *New England Journal of Medicine*, November 18, 1971.

Krauthammer, Charles, "The ethics of human manufacture," *The New Republic*, May 4, 1987.

"On the frontiers of medicine: control of life," *Life*, September 10, 1965.

McLaren, Anne, "Can we diagnose genetic disease in pre-embryos?" *New Scientist*, December 10, 1987.

McLuhan, Marshall, and George Leonard, "The future of sex," *Look*, July 25, 1967.

Muller, Hermann J., "Human evolution by voluntary choice of germ plasm," *Science*, September 8, 1961.

Novak, Michael, "Buying & selling babies: limitations on the marketplace," *Commonweal*, July 17, 1987.

Ramsey, Paul, "Shall we 'reproduce'? Part I. The medical ethics of in vitro fertilization," *Journal of the American Medical Association*, June 5, 1972.

_____, "Shall we 'reproduce'? Part II. Rejoinders and future forecast," *Journal of the American Medical Association*, June 12, 1972.

Rothman, Barbara Katz, "How science is redefining parenthood," *Ms.*, July/August 1982.

Vines, Gail, "New insights into early embryos," *New Scientist*, July 9, 1987.

Will, George, "Discretionary killing," *Newsweek*, September 20, 1976.

Wolfensberger, Wolf, "Common assets of mentally retarded people that are not commonly acknowledged," *Mental Retardation*, April 1988.

INDEX